STAFF DEVELOPMENT NURSING SECRETS

STAFF DEVELOPMENT NURSING SECRETS

Kristen L. O'Shea, MS, RN
Team Leader
Clinical Education
Wellspan Health
York, Pennsylvania

HANLEY & BELFUS, INC. / Philadelphia

Publisher: HANLEY & BELFUS, INC.
Medical Publishers
210 South 13th Street
Philadelphia, PA 19107
(215) 546-7293; 800-962-1892
FAX (215) 790-9330
Web site: http://www.hanleyandbelfus.com

Disclaimer: This book is not intended to be prescriptive, but rather offers the collective wisdom of nursing staff development educators. Although the information in this book has been carefully reviewed for accuracy, neither the authors nor the editor nor the publisher can accept any legal responsibility for any errors. Neither the publisher nor the editor makes any warranty, expressed or implied, with respect to the material contained herein.

Library of Congress Control Number: 2002106245

STAFF DEVELOPMENT NURSING SECRETS ISBN 1-56053-525-3

Last digit is the print number: 9 8 7 6 5 4 3 2 1

CONTENTS

CONTRIBUTORS

Roxanne Amerson, MSN, RN
Associate Degree Nursing Instructor, Tri-County Technical College, Pendleton, South Carolina

Daryl Boucher, RN, MSN, EMT-P
Faculty, Department of Nursing and Allied Health, Northern Maine Technical College; Emergency Department, Aroostook Medical Center, Presque Isle, Maine

Kenneth R. Bowman, RN, MS
Staff Educator, Clinical Information Systems, Department of Professional Education and Development, Lancaster General Hospital, Lancaster, Pennsylvania

Jean M. Bulmer, MSN, RNC
Manager, Center for Education and Staff Development, Hamot Medical Center, Erie, Pennsylvania

Diann C. Cooper, MSN, RNC
Staff Development Specialist, Center for Education and Staff Development, Hamot Medical Center, Erie, Pennsylvania

Cynthia Crockett, MSN, RN
Nursing Education Specialist, Clinical and Patient Education Department, Mayo Clinic Hospital, Phoenix, Arizona

Belinda Curtis, BSN, RN, BC
Nursing Education Specialist, Clinical and Patient Education Department, Mayo Clinic Hospital, Phoenix, Arizona

Linda L. Grasmick, PhD, RN
Clinical Practice and Education Specialist, Children's Hospital of the King's Daughters, Norfolk, Virginia

Connie H. Gutshall, MS, RN, CNA
Director of Clinical Services, Women's and Children's Services, York Hospital-Wellspan Health, York, Pennsylvania

Ann W. Hood, EdD, RN
Director, Center for Nursing Education and Research, Baylor University Medical Center, Dallas, Texas

John L. LaBrie, BSN, RN
Director of Education, Northern Maine Medical Center, Fort Kent, Maine

Kristen L. O'Shea, MS, RN
Team Leader, Clinical Education, Wellspan Health, York, Pennsylvania

Barbara L. Paterson, PhD, RN
Professor, University of British Columbia School of Nursing; Nursing Scholar, Vancouver Hospital and Health Sciences Center, Vancouver, British Columbia, Canada

Cheryl B. Robinson, RN, BSN, MSN
Assistant Professor of Nursing, West Virginia University, Parkersburg, West Virginia

Linda S. Smith, MS, DSN, RN
Assistant Professor of Nursing, Oregon Health and Science University School of Nursing, Klamath Falls, Oregon

Sandra L. Spangenberg, RN, BSN
Manager, Nursing Education, Department of Employee and Organizational Development, Aurora Health Care, Milwaukee, Wisconsin

Rebecca Wilson MSN, RN, C
Nursing Education Specialist, Clinical and Patient Education Department, Mayo Clinic Hospital, Phoenix, Arizona

Angela C. Wolff, MSN, RN
Continuing Education Coordinator, Registered Nurses Association of British Columbia, Vancouver, British Columbia, Canada

PREFACE

What a wonderful experience it has been to create this book. I guessed that it would be professionally gratifying, but I never expected the personal friendships and camaraderie that would result. The contributors to this book come from across the U.S. and Canada. We have communicated primarily via e-mail, a medium that has provided us with a way to contact one another frequently and to share our ideas and experiences. Therefore, each chapter is a compilation of the vast experience of this very talented and committed group of staff development educators. My thanks and respect go to each and every contributor of this book.

Staff development work has no boundaries, and we are involved in many different aspects of health care and an infinite number of projects. Therefore, this book is by no means comprehensive. Instead, it is intended simply to answer the questions of staff development educators as they develop in their roles. It contains advice and nuggets to assist in tackling the daily challenges of our work.

Good educators can make a difference. Instead of impacting individual patients directly, we influence the outcomes of all who are touched by the people we have taught. We should use that power and anticipate and welcome the opportunities to make a difference.

I would like to acknowledge the help and support of my colleagues and family. Linda Scheetz, the Nursing Secrets Series® editor, and my publisher, Linda Belfus, have been incredibly supportive and helpful. Many thanks to the Education Services team at Wellspan Health. You do make a difference! Special thanks to Amy Gotwalt, the comma queen, for proofreading and insight, and to Diane Sargeant, for supporting me all the way. Thanks to Carol Pritchett for patience and administrative support. To my husband, Tom, and children, Kelly, Molly, and Brian, thank you for your support and love. To Fabian, our foreign exchange student from Italy, thank you for cooking! And finally, thank you to my Mom and Dad, for always modeling the importance of continuous learning, creative thinking, and humor. I am grateful for those values.

Kristen L. O'Shea, RN, MS

I. State of the Practice

1. NURSING STAFF DEVELOPMENT AND HEALTH CARE TODAY

Kristen L. O'*Shea*, MS, RN

1. Define nursing staff development.

Nursing staff development describes the formal and informal learning activities that support nurses in their roles within an organization. Currently these learning activities come in many different formats. They may be instructor-led classes or self-directed computer modules. They may be held within a hospital or extended-care facility or outside the organization. Some staff development activities may even be done within the comfort of one's own home, as a nurse sits in front of the family computer.

Traditionally, nursing staff development has included such activities as orientation and preceptor workshops, life support classes, electrocardiogram (EKG) classes, and inservices about new equipment. Today, however, the staff development educator also may teach non-nurses who support clinical functions, provide inspiring leadership development offerings, and influence system-wide goals through various projects and initiatives.

There are many different ways to disseminate knowledge. Computers and two-way video technology have provided new avenues to explore. Indeed, these are exciting times for personnel in nursing staff development.

2. Is nursing staff development a specialty?

Absolutely. Gone are the days when an aging nurse with excellent bedside skills becomes the "inservice nurse." Education specialists need specific knowledge and skills to provide staff development offerings (see Chapters 2 and 4).

The American Nurses Association recognizes staff development as a specialty. In addition, the American Nurses Credentialing Center (ANCC) certifies nurses in nursing continuing education (CE)/staff development through a process that verifies experience and tests knowledge via a certification exam. Additional information about this and other credentialing exams can be found at the ANCC website, nursingworld.org/ancc, or by writing to the ANCC at 600 Maryland Avenue, SW, Suite 100 West, Washington, DC 20024-2571.

3. Where do specialists in nursing staff development work?

Generally you think of staff development specialists as working within the traditional setting of the acute care hospital. Educators also work in long-term care facilities, home care, and outpatient settings as well as within nursing agencies. They may work in a centralized system-wide education department or for a service line, nursing department, or clinical department. A recent request on an nursing staff development listserve yielded the following list of centralized department within which nursing staff development educators work:

- Department of Education and Professional Development
- Education and Consulting
- Education and Development
- Education and Training
- Education Department or Education Services
- Educational Effectiveness and Learning

- Educational Resources in Health Care
- Center for Organizational Development
- Clinical and Patient Education
- Employee and Organizational Development
- Health Professions Continuing Education
- Human Resources Strategic Learning Center
- Human Resources Center for Training and Education
- Organization-wide Development and Education
- Performance Improvement and Education

4. What titles are given to nurses who work in staff development?

- Staff development specialist
- Education specialist
- Staff development coordinator
- Inservice instructor
- Education and development specialist
- Employee development coordinator
- Nurse educator
- Clinical resource supervisor
- Staff development educator
- Clinical educator

5. What is the difference between a clinical nurse specialist and an education specialist?

Definitely some aspects of the two roles are similar. The clinical nurse specialist has a master's degree and has been educated to care for the most complex patients. The focus of the clinical nurse specialist is divided among six primary roles: expert clinician, educator, change agent, researcher, care manager, and consultant. The focus of an education specialist is divided between two primary roles: educator and change agent. A master's degree is not always required for the education specialist.

6. How long has nursing staff development been around?

Nursing staff development has been around since Florence Nightingale, who believed that lifelong learning was an important part of nursing practice. She told her students that nurses must never consider themselves "finished" because "there is no end in what we may be learning every day."[2] Formal nursing staff development offerings are noted in the literature as early as 1895. Nurses have a long history of acknowledging the need for ongoing education and skill development.

7. During the 1970s, it seemed that nursing staff development clearly reported to nursing. Now it seems more "system-focused." What happened?

During the health care changes in the late 1980s and 1990s, hospitals were restructured. Staff development educators across the country found themselves changing roles. In some cases, nursing staff development stayed within the department of nursing. However, others found themselves working within departments of human resources or organizational development. Some educators found themselves aligned with service lines. As more and more hospitals became part of larger systems, the development of system-wide education departments became more common. Many specialists in nursing staff development are responsible for education of health care providers across multiple sites. Some sites are miles apart. Unquestionably the past decade has brought many changes for specialists in nursing staff development. Our roles keep getting bigger and bigger, but in many cases, our numbers are getting smaller and smaller.

8. What current trends in health care are affecting staff development?

Undeniably, recruitment and retention of nurses and diminishing revenues are key issues. The volume of activities designed to enhance recruitment and retention of nurses is up, while at the same time the available resources to do the added work is down. This situation has caused many education departments to change their priorities. In some cases, existing programming has been cut to provide more frequent and flexible orientation and required education.

A vicious cycle emerges as the shortage of nurses causes more nurses to leave the profession. Health care organizations make increasing use of agency nursing staff to fill gaps. Some hospitals recruit foreign nurses to fill positions. This strategy presents a unique orientation challenge (see Chapter 15). Understaffing results in burnout and decreased morale. Patient and physician satisfaction also suffer in units that experience high vacancy rates and high turnover. Getting nurses to educational offerings becomes nearly impossible because of understaffing.

Concerns about patient safety in view of the nursing shortage and the Institute of Medicine's report about health care errors have placed nursing staff development educators in an important position. A renewed emphasis on ensuring staff competency and providing current information is evident. The trick is to find new ways to reach nurses who are unable to leave their busy units.

9. How does the Joint Commission for Accreditation of Healthcare Organizations (JCAHO) affect the staff development educator?

The JCAHO is one of the accrediting bodies that may visit your organization. Their mission is to improve the quality and safety of health care provided to the public. A number of JCAHO standards support education within an organization. The human resources standards require competency assessment, orientation, and encouragement and availability of self-development and learning.The JCAHO may ask staff: "Are you able to get to educational offerings? What offerings have you been able to attend this year?" (For more information about JCAHO requirements, see Chapter 20.)

10. How do business trends influence the work of specialists in nursing staff development?

Luckily a business emphasis on education has followed the "restructuring/downsizing" patterns of the 1990s. Key business leaders repeatedly have shown that the key to success in business is nurturing vital human resources. Tom Peters, a well-known leadership guru, summarizes the philosophy: "Brains are in; heavy lifting is out. That's the essential nature of the new, knowledge-based economy. Therefore, the development of knowledge is close to job No. 1 for most corporations."[1]

Another important trend in business has been rapid development of "e-learning"—that is, learning activities available through electronic means (e.g., computer-based training, conferences via two-way video equipment). Large businesses worldwide have found that e-learning cuts education time and enhances individual development. Health care organizations are also beginning to embrace this concept.

11. What is a learning organization?

During the early 1990s, Peter Senge provided the vision of a learning organization in *The Fifth Discipline*.[3] A learning organization continually expands its capacity to create its own future. According to Senge, five learning disciplines promote lifelong learning and study:

1. **Personal mastery:** expanding personal capacity as well as creating an organization that is committed to encouraging employees to develop themselves.
2. **Mental models:** taking time to reflect on and improve the "internal pictures" of the world.
3. **Shared vision:** building a sense of commitment to a shared vision.
4. **Team learning:** developing thinking skills so that groups of people see the collective knowledge and ability of the group as greater than the sum of the individual members' talents.
5. **Systems thinking:** a way of viewing and understanding the interrelationships of everything around us.

Subsequent books[4,5] by Senge provide resources and practical suggestions related to building and maintaining a learning organization.

12. What are CKOs and CLOs?

CKOs are chief knowledge officers; CLOs are chief learning officers. Both are senior administrators responsible for the process of disseminating the vast amount of information and knowledge that is necessary in the current market. This new role is appearing in businesses and hospital systems across the country. The development of such a role signals that organizations are beginning to understand the importance of knowledge and information.

13. How can staff development educators affect recruitment and retention efforts?

The literature demonstrates clearly the important role of staff development educators in efforts to attract and keep nurses. Staff development educators can affect recruitment and retention daily through involvement in strong programming. Across the country, orientation and internship programs are being retooled and expanded. Critical care units that have not hired graduate nurses since the late 1980s (the last nursing shortage) are now counting on internships to provide competent nurses. The important role of the preceptor in facilitating the orientation of new nurses has emerged once again, as evidenced by a resurgence of preceptor education and reward programs. Nurse refresher courses are cropping up across the country as a means of supporting the return of nurses who have taken a break from their careers.

In addition, staff development educators affect the level of satisfaction and morale among nurses as they try to support continued work in their facilities. Offerings to help nurses do their jobs better, keep on top of current trends and motivate continued love for the profession assist in retention efforts. Fellowship programs within hospitals offer nurses an opportunity to "try out" new specialties without leaving their departments or hospitals. Through fellowships, a nurse who has been in her area for a year or two is offered an opportunity to choose a new specialty and "try it out" for a week with pay. This practice promotes individual development and retention of staff.

Nurse educators also may be involved in clinical ladder development. Clinical ladders are designed to promote professional development of bedside nurses. Without a clinical ladder it may not be possible for nurses to advance or seek promotion without leaving bedside nursing. A clinical ladder provides the opportunity for promotion and rewards the nurse's depth of practice and involvement within the unit and organization (see Chapter 22).

14. Why does the current health care system seem so crazy?

Nurses are busier now than ever. They face the prospect of a growing aging population, financial challenges, new competition, nursing shortages, huge medical advances that shorten and intensify patient stays, and, finally, smarter (and perhaps more demanding) patients.

Tim Porter O'Grady recently reflected on the fact that most nurses grew up in the Industrial Age. We worked hard and learned a lot in nursing school. We took copious notes and memorized everything. But now, in the Information Age, everything has changed. We are barraged with information constantly, and all the while we are trying to be nurses as we always have been. O'Grady suggests that nurses need to change the way they do business to manage information differently. We need to help nurses learn to focus on what is important.

After finishing an interview with Albert Einstein, a reporter asked for the famous scientist's phone number in case he needed more information as he worked on the article. Einstein had to look up his own phone number in the directory. The reporter was flabbergasted. Einstein explained that he needed to know lots of information but could always look up his own phone number. This strategy saved room for other information. As we look at our crazy times, we need to help nurses rethink the way in which they perform their jobs and give them resources and references to enhance performance.

15. How else can staff development specialists help nurses cope with the current state of health care?

Consider incorporating stress management and other types of personal development offerings into education sessions. Offerings on topics such as diffusing emotionally charged situations and communicating with patients are important and often attractive to staff. As a matter of fact, at our hospital, the offering on diffusing emotionally charged situations has a waiting list! Obviously nurses need tools to deal with the incredible pressures of health care. Staff development educators can suggest possible ways to deal with the rapid change and stress that nurses now face.

16. What are the greatest challenges for staff development/education departments?

The current reality is that there are fewer educators and less time and money for education, even though the need for education is greater than ever. Given new technologies, nurses returning to practice who need refreshing, and nurses recruited from foreign countries, your job is cut out for you. The challenge is to do more with less. You need to find new ways of providing education and to be as flexible as possible.

17. What can I do to stay sane?

It is absolutely necessary to model behaviors related to stress management. Take care of yourself. Eat well and exercise. Find your passions, and make sure that you engage in activities that you enjoy. I often tell nurses that the beauty of nursing is that you can do so many different things because of the infinite possibilities in the profession. It is possible, therefore, to find your passion.

Have fun! Humor is critical. Build humor into the educational offerings that you provide. Build relationships, and connect with people. Make time for a balance between work and home. These strategies will help you cope with the crazy times that we are facing.

BIBLIOGRAPHY

1. Peters T: The Pursuit of Wow! New York, Random House, 1994.
2. Schuyler CB: Florence Nightingale. In Nightingale F: Notes of Nursing (Commemorative Edition, with introduction by Barbara Stevens Barnum and commentaries by contemporary nursing leaders). Philadelphia, J.B. Lippincott, 1992, p 11.
3. Senge PM: The Fifth Discipline. New York, Doubleday, 1990.
4. Senge PM, et al: The Fifth Discipline Fieldbook. New York, Doubleday, 1994.
5. Senge PM, et al: The Dance of Change. New York, Doubleday, 1999.

2. ROLES OF THE STAFF DEVELOPMENT EDUCATOR

Linda L. Grasmick, PhD, RN

1. The role of the staff development educator is to plan and teach educational programs. What else is there?

As part of an institution's nursing leadership team, staff development educators are often called on to fulfill a wide variety of functions. In addition, the actual process of providing education may require the instructor to assume many different roles.

Traditionally, the staff development role has included education, management, consultation, and research activities. Recently, however, the American Nurses Association (ANA) revised this concept slightly. The ANA used the expression "nursing professional development" to encompass all types of educational programs that a nurse may attend to maintain competence, enhance professional practice, and support the achievement of career goals. Nursing professional development thus incorporates the distinct but overlapping domains of staff development, continuing education, and academic education (particularly beyond the level of basic preparation). The six roles of the nursing professional development educator, as described by the ANA, provide a starting point from which to base a discussion of the many functions of the nursing staff development educator (see table below).

Six Aspects of the Staff Development Educator's Role

ROLE	KEY POINTS	EXAMPLES
1. Educator	Provides educational programs for staff (assesses, plans, presents, evaluates, and documents) Learners may be nurses or non-nurses Does not typically include patient education, but job expectations may vary because of need for educational expertise and availability	Staff orientation New equipment and procedure inservices Clinical practice updates and reviews Local or regional conference programs
2. Facilitator	Helps others to identify learning needs and resources Arranges and organizes programs taught by others Serves on committees that plan, solve problems, or direct organizational activities	Maintaining resource library for staff use Arranging new equipment in-service taught by company representative Conducting team-building exercises to promote work group harmony and effectiveness Conducting literature search for committee or work group
3. Change agent	Identifies and initiates needed change Helps others to adopt change and to adapt to change in health care environment Change may occur at unit, institutional, regional, national, or international level	Developing new policies and competencies Teaching staff about needed practice changes Helping staff to solve problems as they implement changes in practice

Table continued on following page

Six Aspects of the Staff Development Educator's Role (Continued)

	KEY POINTS	EXAMPLES
...nt	May be formal or informal Advises individuals or groups about educational issues Helps others with problem definition and resolution	Providing advice and/or information to help staff solve clinical practice problem Helping another unit or facility to plan or evaluate an educational program
5. Researcher	Conducts research and/or promotes conduct of research by others Disseminates research findings Promotes research utilization May relate to either clinical practice or educational topics	Basing educational programs on current research findings Teaching staff about research processes Serving as member of research team Publishing/presenting knowledge developed through research or evaluation activities
6. Leader	May include activities commonly associated with management roles Strives for congruence between educational activities and institutional mission and goals Demonstrates support for professional organizations and excellence in professional practice and development	Managing educational budget Mentoring less experienced colleagues Participating in professional organizations Role-modeling desirable qualities and actions

2. What is included in the educator role?

The educator role includes most of the activities that first come to mind when people think about a staff development role. It includes the planning and teaching of nursing educational programs, activities that are discussed in depth throughout this book. However, the educator role also includes a few activities that may be less obvious. For example, a novice nurse educator may be surprised by the challenge of teaching non-nursing personnel, such as secretaries and housekeepers. In such situations, the staff development educator must first research both the job requirements and the learning abilities and preferences of the personnel before planning educational programs. Non-nursing personnel and professional nursing staff may have quite different needs and preferences.

Educators also evaluate the effectiveness of their programs. This activity requires not only knowledge of evaluation processes but also the willingness to make the extra effort to collect and analyze data long after teaching the program. Although it may be tempting to skip the evaluation and to focus instead on upcoming programs, only a high-quality evaluation can help the educator draw valid conclusions about a program's effectiveness and needs for changes or additional follow-up.

Finally, educators maintain records of the programs that they provide. Such records typically include a list of attendees and faculty as well as a summary of the learning needs assessment, course content, teaching strategies and materials, and program evaluation. People may need these records to support applications for jobs, schools, or professional certification. Institutions may use the records to evaluate employee performance and to demonstrate that they have met the standards of regulatory and accreditation agencies.

3. Does the educator role include patient education?

Technically speaking, the function of staff development does not include patient education. In the interests of efficiency, however, the line between staff education and patient education is sometimes blurred in the real world. In particular, when educational resources are scarce, staff members may do "double-duty." Some institutions have roles such as "clinical nurse specialist" or "unit educator" that combine many functions, including both staff and patient education. As another example, cardiopulmonary resuscitation instructors may teach classes for patients and the general public as well as for professionals. Finally, a hospital may combine its staff development educators and patient educators within one administrative department to consolidate educational resources and promote the sharing of expertise and coordination of effort. These are examples of how the roles of staff educator and patient educator can overlap, even though they are two distinct functions.

4. What does it mean to be a facilitator?

Facilitators help people accomplish goals and keep systems running smoothly. This aspect of the staff development role includes many activities that occur behind the scenes and that may go unnoticed, even though they can be quite time-consuming. For example, an educator may make arrangements for a guest speaker and then ensure that the speaker has the resources needed to make the class a success (e.g., classroom, audiovisual equipment, refreshments). The educator does not actually teach the class but facilitates the educational process. Staff development educators also act as facilitators when they help staff identify their own learning needs, direct them to appropriate resources, and promote the processes of life-long learning.

Participation in committees and other work groups provides another example of how educators can serve as facilitators. Educators often have knowledge and skills useful for group work, such as knowledge of organizational processes and ability to find and organize information. Other members of the group with clinical, but not organizational, expertise may look to the educator to help keep the group productive and on track.

5. How can I become a good facilitator?

Good facilitators are usually popular with their colleagues and in high demand by people looking to form a work team. Here are a few tips on how to develop your skills as a facilitator:

1. Learn as much as you can about your work environment. Know the proper procedures for obtaining supplies and processing paperwork. Become the expert on "where to find things" and "how to get things done."
2. Learn to use library (and Internet) resources. Be the person who can get information quickly.
3. Identify people to whom you can turn when you need help. Make friends with secretaries and other members of the support staff. Know the names of people in other departments. Maintain a list of useful telephone numbers. These resources can be lifesavers and help you to help others.
4. Be visible and available. Ask people how they are doing and whether there is anything they need.
5. If you are unable to fulfill someone's needs, be honest. Raising false hopes and unrealistic expectations leads to disappointment later. However, if you can help people locate other possible resources, they will still be happy that they sought your help.
6. Set limits. Good facilitators help other people do their jobs; they do not do other people's jobs for them. Your help should allow others to experience the satisfaction of accomplishment, not take that joy from them.
7. Document the assistance that you provide whenever possible. At least be sure that key people (e.g., your immediate supervisor) are aware of this aspect of your practice and the contributions that you make to other people's projects. You may want to prepare a monthly (or quarterly) report that includes all of your activities, not just your primary responsibilities.

6. How do staff development educators act as change agents?

The purpose behind most staff development programs is to change the behavior of the participants— to help them practice in new and better ways. Thus, through their teaching, staff development educators change practice and improve patient care. In addition, staff members frequently turn to educators to help them answer questions and resolve problems that arise during the process of change. Educators serve as resources during the change process, helping the staff to adopt new methods of care delivery and to adapt to changes in the work environment.

Educators also act as change agents when they participate in the development of policies and competencies, and when they serve on committees that establish institutional or professional priorities and standards. Through interactions with staff and monitoring of patient care (for learning needs assessment and program evaluation), educators can identify practice issues that need attention. Participation in institutional committees and professional organizations provides avenues through which the educator can address such issues.

7. What exactly is a nurse consultant?

In *Nurses as Consultants*,[6] Susan Norwood defines nursing consultation as "working with individuals or groups to help them resolve actual or potential problems related to the health status of clients or health care delivery." In other words, nurse consultants help their colleagues solve work-related problems with the ultimate goal of improving patient care. Consultants assess situations, diagnose and define problems, and make recommendations for how problems may be solved. The person who requested the consultation (the consultee) is then free to accept, modify, or completely reject the recommendations provided by the consultant. This is a key point in the consultation process: the consultee retains ownership of the situation. The job of the consultant is not to take command but to provide the consultee with options from which to choose.

8. Describe the process of consultation.

Consultation may be a relatively small and informal process, as when a staff nurse seeks advice on how to handle a specific clinical situation. The consultation comes and goes in a matter of minutes. On the other hand, the consultation may be quite large and formal, as when an expert educator is asked to assess a hospital's entire educational program and make recommendations for improvement. From beginning to end, such a consultation may take several months. Although on the surface these two examples may seem quite different, both conform to the same basic process, which Norwood describes as consisting of five phases:

1. Gaining entry
2. Problem identification
3. Action planning
4. Evaluation
5. Disengagement

During the first phase of gaining entry, the consultant and consultee become acquainted with each other to determine whether they want to pursue a relationship. Assuming that they do, the parties define their relationship and establish their expectations of one another. In the more modest example above, the staff nurse and the educator probably already have a relationship; to gain entry, the educator only needs to be available. In the larger example, the consultant and consultee probably have several preliminary discussions about the project before formally establishing their relationship in a written contract.

In the problem identification phase, the consultant collects and analyzes information, diagnoses the problem, and presents the findings to the consultee. It is vital at this stage to secure the support of the consultee for the conclusions drawn so that the next phase—action planning—can be done collaboratively. During the action-planning phase, the consultant and consultee set goals and plan interventions. After helping the consultee to implement the interventions (if help is needed), the consultant evaluates both the effectiveness of the interventions and the overall process of consultation. In the final phase of disengagement, both parties acknowledge the end of the collaboration and the consultee's preparedness to continue without further help from the consultant.

9. What special skills or qualities do I need to be a good consultant?

- Technical skills (diagnostic and problem-solving skills)
- Human process skills (communication and interpersonal skills)
- Broad knowledge base
- Certain personal attributes
- Professionalism

Consultants need the technical skills to gather and analyze information for adequate assessment and correct diagnosis of the situation. They also need the ability to conceptualize the problem appropriately and to develop goals and possible solutions. Human process skills, or "people skills," are also an important asset for nurse consultants. Communication and interpersonal skills enable the consultant to establish and maintain productive relationships and to keep the consultation process moving in a positive direction. Nurse consultants also benefit from a broad base of knowledge about both human and organizational behavior. For example, a knowledge of change theory, systems theory, group dynamics, adult learning theory, and conflict resolution help the consultant to understand the environment and to work successfully within it.

As for the personal qualities required for successful consultation, Norwood emphasizes the need for consultants to be able to convey a sense of empathy, warmth, respect, acceptance, and concern. She also emphasizes the need for flexibility along with tolerance for ambiguity and lack of total control. The subject of the consultation may be quite complex, and the interests of many parties may need to be considered. In addition, consultants share the responsibility for problem resolution with the consultee and must be prepared for the possibility that the consultee will choose not to follow through with all of the recommended actions.

Finally, Norwood discusses the key professional attributes needed by nurse consultants. She emphasizes the need for good judgment and clear understanding of the responsibilities and obligations of the consultant. She also emphasizes the need to recognize one's limitations and to continue the process of growth and development.

Note the compatibility between the skills and qualities needed by nurse consultants and other aspects of the staff development role. Honing your skills as a consultant also helps in many other areas of your practice.

10. Do I have to do research?

Many nurses balk at the thought of incorporating a research component into their roles. Some may be intimidated by statistical analysis. Others may find the process of conducting research to be painstaking and boring. Most of us have trouble with finding time in busy schedules for one more activity—particularly for a project that may not have an obvious and immediate benefit. Regardless of the reasons, research is an aspect of staff development practice that often is placed near the bottom of the priority list.

However, it is crucial that staff development educators participate in the research process. Educators based in a practice setting can provide vital links between the research processes that generate nursing knowledge and the clinical processes that utilize such knowledge. Without linkages to clinical practice, knowledge development can become irrelevant and impractical—and without linkages to the ever-evolving nursing knowledge base, clinical practice can become ineffective and inefficient. Staff development educators can facilitate the work of both clinical staff and researchers by ensuring that neither group works in isolation.

If you feel a bit intimidated by the thought of adding a research component to your practice, it may help to define the term broadly to include all of the activities involved in the development, dissemination, and utilization of knowledge. By considering each separately and in a little more detail, you may be surprised at how much research you already do.

11. How can I help in the development of new research-based knowledge?

Tuohig and Oleson[7] discuss several ways that staff development educators can help encourage and facilitate the research process in the clinical arena:

1. Brainstorming to generate research ideas and questions
2. Collaborating with other disciplines
3. Providing education for staff about research topics and resources
4. Assisting in data collection
5. Helping people to locate and utilize resources (e.g., librarians, statisticians, computer experts)
6. Arranging for statistical analysis
7. Organizing meetings or discussions to keep everyone up to date on ongoing projects.

Staff development educators can either conduct research themselves or help others conduct research. If you are new to the practice of research, helping others is a great way to get started.

12. How can I help others to conduct research?

Whether the principal investigator for a research project works regularly in the clinical setting or is from an outside academic institution, he or she may need help working within the hospital system and with the nursing staff. The researcher may need education about the clinical unit's policies and customary practices, and the unit staff may need education about the research project's goals and procedures. Educators based in a clinical setting are in a perfect position to facilitate the research process in this way.

Providing education for the staff about research processes is another way to promote nursing research within your institution and to participate in the process yourself. Staff may need to learn more about searching and reviewing the literature or writing proposals and reports. They also may need information about your employer's institutional review board or assistance in locating resources that can help them plan research projects (e.g., statisticians). Once again, staff development educators are often in a good position to help the staff access both the informational and human resources that they need to conduct studies.

13. What if I want to develop my own research project? Where do I start?

To begin conducting your own research, pay attention to the questions that arise in your day-to-day practice. Are there clinical questions for which the literature does not provide adequate answers? Are you making changes in your practice that could (and should) be evaluated with pre- and post-change measurements? How do you evaluate your educational programs? Do your program evaluations show that certain teaching methods work better than others? Are there certain aspects of clinical care or educational practice that particularly interest you?

As you think about such questions, consider how you may go about answering them. What kind of data should you collect? What problems might you encounter if you were to set up a little research project? Discuss your interests, questions, and concerns with colleagues. Do any of them share your interests? Are any of them interested in working with you on a project to explore or evaluate a specific topic in more detail?

Sometimes it helps to link your project with the institution's performance improvement (or quality assurance) program. Performance improvement staff members can provide a structure and a format for your project as well as access to people who can help you with data collection and analysis. There also may be a nursing research committee or similar group that you can join (or consult) to help get started. Faculty members at local schools of nursing also may be interested in working with you and helping you to get started.

14. Do you have any more suggestions on how to get started?

1. Start small. Small projects, such as the evaluation of a single educational program or a single change in practice, give you a chance to develop skills without overextending yourself. As your skill and comfort levels grow, you can move on to larger and more complex projects.

2. Select a topic that is a routine aspect of your practice. This strategy keeps you focused on the topic and helps keep your research grounded in real-life practice.

3. Nurture your relationships with people who may be able to help you—even if you are not currently working on a project.

4. Read articles and books, and attend conferences related to research, particularly local conferences. Join your local chapter of Sigma Theta Tau. This strategy keeps you inspired and helps you meet colleagues with similar interests.

5. Create a file folder or notebook of materials related to your topic (or topics) of interest. Create another file or notebook of materials related to the research process. You also may find it helpful to keep a journal of ideas that you can review periodically.

6. Talk about your interests with anyone who will listen. Talking about them keeps your thought processes moving forward—and sometimes, talking helps you to find supportive colleagues.

7. Finally, just do it. Your first few attempts may not work out the way you hoped. If the projects are small, you have little to lose. But with each project, regardless of the outcome, you will learn valuable lessons for the future.

15. How can I help with the dissemination of research-based knowledge?

The easiest way to become involved in the research process is to help with the dissemination of the knowledge developed through research. Knowledge is of little use to your staff if they never learn about it. You probably disseminate a lot of research-based knowledge already as you teach classes and keep your staff up to date on the latest developments in nursing science. How many of the following activities do you already do? Are there a few activities on the list that perhaps you should try?

1. Base your educational programs, policies, and competencies on current research findings whenever possible. Cite the research and discuss its applicability to practice with the staff to promote an awareness of its use.
2. Post relevant research articles for your staff to read (monthly or quarterly). If you think that they may have difficulty in interpreting parts of the article or applying the results to their practice, provide a brief synopsis of the key points along with the article.
3. Start a journal club that meets periodically to review current research articles.
4. Ensure that your hospital library subscribes to nursing journals that include research relevant to your practice. You also may want to subscribe yourself or purchase a subscription for your department.
5. Create file folders, drawers, or notebooks of relevant literature as you find it. Create your own mini-library of material most relevant to your work. It will then be easy to access later, when you need it.
6. Invite colleagues at your hospital to present their projects (large or small) as inservices for the staff. Organize a poster fair, or arrange for brief presentations of the work during Nurses' Week. This approach not only helps to disseminate the information but also provides your colleagues with positive reinforcement and encouragement.
7. Publish or present your work and/or help your colleagues do the same. Submit an abstract to create a poster for a professional conference. Many nurses hesitate because their projects are relatively modest in size or scope. However, many conferences welcome the inclusion of real-life practice projects that demonstrate the usefulness of research-based knowledge or that illustrate new approaches to solving common problems.

16. How can I help with the utilization of research-based knowledge?

The final step in the research process is utilization. Utilization validates the results of the research and gives a purpose to all of the work that went into it—the purpose of being used by nurses to improve their practice and provide better patient care. Mottola[5] identified three major barriers to research utilization and suggested strategies that staff development educators can use to overcome those barriers.

1. The first barrier is the **limited availability of research findings**. In fact, research relevant to your areas of interest may exist, but it may be published in obscure journals or written in ways that make it difficult for the average nurse to interpret and apply. The staff development educator can help overcome this barrier through the active dissemination of research-based knowledge, as previously discussed. Helping the staff to locate and interpret current literature is an important first step in the research utilization process.
2. The second barrier to research utilization is **the knowledge and attitudes of many nurses**. Few nurses receive more than a cursory introduction to research processes or findings in their basic education programs, and many aspects of actual nursing practice are based on tradition rather than cited research results. At the practice level, nursing is not a profession with a history and tradition of risk-taking, change-agency, and research-based practice. Once again, some of the previously mentioned activities can be used by the staff development educator to further the staff's knowledge of and interest in research and its applicability to practice. Educators can help staff to locate and evaluate relevant literature and can provide a positive role model by openly citing the research used to prepare classes and to develop policies and competencies.
3. The third barrier is **poor environmental support**. Clinical institutions focused on the provision of patient care may not provide an environment conducive to research utilization,

which requires (among other things) time, money, and cultural support for nurses who dare to initiate changes in practice. It may be unrealistic to expect to change an environment overnight. Over time, however, an educator can influence the culture of a particular department or institution by consistently demonstrating the value of research-based practice and by supporting the efforts of fellow nurses to improve practice through research utilization. Personal experience validates this assertion. The case study that concludes this chapter helped change the attitudes and sense of empowerment of many nurses and had a significant effect on unit culture.

17. What leadership activities are commonly done by staff development educators?

The ANA[3] describes the leadership role as "providing and supporting organizational and administrative structures to achieve departmental and organizational goals." This aspect of the staff development role includes many of the activities commonly associated with management roles, such as preparing and managing a budget and supervising personnel. It may surprise some educators to find themselves expected to perform such duties, but they come hand-in-hand with managing an educational program and/or providing leadership for an education department. Educators must frequently determine the costs of the programs that they provide and are expected to manage competently the resources (money, equipment, and personnel) that they are given.

Staff development educators also are expected to provide leadership by actively demonstrating support for the institution. You can demonstrate your support by ensuring that educational programs are congruent with the mission and goals of your employer and by role-modeling the behaviors desired of all employees. Mentoring less-experienced colleagues and serving as a committee chairman are other ways to provide leadership within your institution.

Outside their employing organization, staff development educators may demonstrate leadership through active participation in professional organizations. Such activities provide a way for the nurse to influence the profession on a regional or national scale. They also provide the nurse with an opportunity to network with colleagues with similar interests. In addition, professional organizations often provide members with high-quality educational programs and materials.

18. Must all staff development educators execute all six of the roles?

Yes and no. It is hard to imagine a successful, experienced staff development educator whose practice does not incorporate all six roles over time. However, at any one time, an individual educator may find that one or two aspects of the role predominate and others fade into the background. A novice educator may engage in few leadership or research behaviors, whereas a more experienced educator may have a role that emphasizes leadership and research more than the other aspects. Needs, responsibilities, resources, and abilities change over time, and the specific implementation of the staff development educator's role must be flexible enough to accommodate the ever-changing health care environment. Chapter 3 addresses in detail many of the factors that influence the nature of specific educator roles.

It is not uncommon, however, for a staff development educator to engage in all six aspects of the role on the same day—or within the scope of a single project. The following case study from the author's personal experience illustrates such a project. At the time, my job title was clinical nurse specialist, a role that included responsibility for staff development in a level-III neonatal intensive care unit (NICU).

CASE STUDY

The simple educational request was made on a Thursday afternoon: Would I please teach the nurses how to use a new IV pump? Because I was unable to meet with the company representative, I was on my own—sitting at a table with a portable IV minipump designed for home insulin infusions, a research article describing 10 cases for which it had been used in neonates, and an owner's manual. Being relatively new in my job and wanting to make a good impression on the medical director, I did my best that afternoon to figure out how we could use the pump to provide a new therapy—continuous insulin infusion—in the NICU. The next morning we got our first patient.

Over the next several months, my role in the continuous insulin infusion project consisted mainly of teaching the staff how to use the pump, solving problems with implementation (such as availability of supplies), advising the staff about the nursing management of specific patients, and promoting productive communication among physicians and nurses. These activities reflect the educational, consultation, facilitation, and change agent roles of the staff development educator. I was assisting the physicians in their efforts to implement a new therapy by educating the nursing staff and facilitating the change process.

However, as time passed and we implemented the new therapy with several patients, I saw a need to assume more of a leadership role. No data were being collected about the effectiveness of this therapy, and I saw a need to evaluate our practice more thoroughly. I also noticed that I was the only staff member who had been personally involved with each and every case for which the therapy had been used. Because the nurses consulted me about using the pump and implementing the therapy, I had been involved with all of the cases and found myself as the person with the most experience in this new therapy. That experience had given me insight that was not shared by other members of the nursing staff or by the physicians, each of whom had dealt only with the one or two patients who had needed the therapy on their watch.

I began to collect data in the form of a series of case studies, adding a research component to the project. As the case study data were analyzed, they formed the basis for future education and for making changes in how we administered continuous insulin infusion therapy. The most dramatic change involved assigning the titration of insulin to the nursing staff; previously each change in the infusion rate had required a written physician's order. This change involved the development of a treatment protocol and intense education for the nursing staff. In addition, assuming responsibility for insulin titration required the nursing staff to assume additional risks in their practice, for which they needed support and encouragement from both nursing and medical colleagues.

Eventually it was time to share the experience and the knowledge gained from it with others. During the course of the project, I had presented the work in progress at two nursing conferences, once as a poster and once as a brief podium presentation. Almost six years after the project was begun, I published an article in a multidisciplinary journal.[4] The article summarized 40 case studies generated over a period of 4 years as well as the titration protocols used and a discussion of the problems encountered. I also included a description of the educational methods used to develop expertise within the nursing staff (serial case study review) and two theoretical models on which my selection of the teaching method was based.

Ultimately the continuous insulin infusion project involved all aspects of the nursing staff development role: education, facilitation, change agency, consultation, research, and leadership. The project resulted in improved patient care and an increased sense of empowerment and pride among the nursing staff. Looking back over my 24 years of nursing practice, most of which has been spent in nursing education, I believe that this project has given me the most satisfaction and greatest sense of pride—and it all began with a simple educational request on a Thursday afternoon.

BIBLIOGRAPHY

1. Abruzzese RS, Yoder-Wise AS: Staff development: Our heritage, our visions. In Abruzzese RS (ed): Nursing Staff Development: Strategies for Success, 2nd ed. St. Louis, Mosby, 1996, pp 3–15.
2. American Nurses Association Council on Continuing Education and Staff Development: Roles and Responsibilities for Nursing Continuing Education and Staff Development Across All Settings. Washington, DC, American Nurses Association, 1992.
3. American Nurses Association: Scope and Standards of Practice for Nursing Professional Development. Washington, DC, American Nurses Association, 2000.
4. Grasmick LL: Continuous insulin infusion for the treatment of hyperglycemia in premature infants. Neonat Pharmacol Q 1:47–54, 1992.
5. Mottola CA: Research utilization and the continuing/staff development educator, J Contin Educ Nurs 27(4):168–175, 1996.
6. Norwood SL: Nurses as Consultants. Menlo Park, CA, Addison-Wesley, 1998.
7. Touhig GM, Oleson KJ: Enhancing clinical nursing research: A vital role for staff development educators. J Contin Educ Nurs 28(4):147–149, 1995.

3. FACTORS THAT AFFECT THE EDUCATOR'S ROLE

Ann W. Hood, EdD, RN

1. What questions does the new educator need to ask?

This book is dedicated to helping educators, new and experienced, prepare to lead the educational effort in their health care setting. As the educator begins the role, several questions need to be asked:

1. *What is my role in this organization?* Even if you have been an educator in another facility, you should clarify your role in this particular organization.

2. *Why did I take this position?* It is one thing to seek out a position in education and entirely another to be "drafted" into doing so. The function of education and teaching others is like any other specialty in nursing and health care: you must put a great deal of effort into what you are doing, learn constantly, and become an expert in the field. Your heart as well as your mind should be focused on the role.

3. *How do I go about assisting education in this organization?* Refer to the other chapters in this book. Particularly if you are new, make this book your constant companion for a while. Assessing education, practicing adult learning principles, and planning/creating a learning environment are large aspects of the role of educator. This knowledge is a step forward.

4. *What is my philosophy of education? What is the philosophy of the organization?* You should be able to communicate your beliefs, attitudes, and values related to education and the process of learning. How congruent is your philosophy with that of your employer? As you read this book, step back and assess the position of your organization in regard to education (see question 2).

5. *What resources do I have to begin, and what do I need?* Resources include physical tools such as books, tables, and visual equipment as well as time (including yours and the time provided by the organization for each staff member), money (the budget for education), and people (who and how many people are dedicated to education). Can you realistically do what is expected with the available resources? (See question 8.)

6. *What can I do to educate myself about being an educator?* There are many books to read and seminars to attend. Perhaps a good course in training the trainer or a community college course in adult education theory would be wise. If you take a position as an educator, it becomes your responsibility to learn as much as you can about the educational process (see question 12).

7. *How should I market myself to the staff?* This question is often ignored. Do not assume that, simply because you are the new educator, the staff will follow your lead in matters of practice or knowledge. Gaining the trust of the staff is probably the most important goal; once you gain their trust, you can begin to influence. Get to know the staff, have one-on-one conversations with staff members throughout the facility, hold focus groups, and talk to managers about their philosophy of staff development and how you can meet their unit's needs. In most healthcare organizations, educators cannot "do it all"; they need a few frontline ambassadors. Building positive relationships is how you get them. This is the beginning of your effort to build credibility as an educator.

8. *How will I make the transition from staff to educator?* One day at a time! Most new roles are at first overwhelming because of the new knowledge and skills required. Take time to ask the questions, get the answers, and develop a plan. Do not simply "jump right in." You will become frustrated. You have accepted a new job for which you need to learn new skills, and sometimes you leave your clinical skills to those who follow. If you try to do it all, the job can become overwhelming.

2. What should I know about the organization's educational philosophy?

- What does the organization believe and practice in relation to education?
- What do administrators see as the responsibility of the organization in educating staff?
- What do the chief executive office and chief nursing officer believe about education?
- How important is education in the life of the organization?
- How much time and money is the hospital willing to invest in staff education?

One-hour staff meetings once a month will not accomplish "development." If no formal, written philosophy is available, take the lead and help the organization create one. Two important clues to how an organization feels about education are the position and function of education in the organization and the budget that supports educational initiatives. Whether formal or informal, all hospitals have a philosophy that communicates how important they believe education is.

3. Why is it important identify the philosophy of the organization?

The educator must ensure that the programs coming from the education department are in alignment with the mission, vision, and goals of the entire organization.

4. How does the setting affect the educator's role?

The setting, defined as type of facility (e.g., acute care, long-term care, day surgery, multiple physician practice, pediatric practice, mental health practice), affects the process of education by identification of the ultimate customer. In acute-care hospitals, the patient is with you for only a few days; staff must be able to complete care within this time frame. In long-term care facilities, however, the requirements of staff are different; therefore, the requirements of educators are different. Education should be planned for the type of setting and the ultimate customer. All settings have specific guidelines and regulations that must be understood by staff and educators. For example, the paper work alone in a transitional care unit is an important learning process.

Setting can affect urgency of education. Information in acute-care hospitals moves at a rapid pace; information is needed yesterday. In other types of facilities, the flow of care and information is paced differently because clients are in the facility for longer periods and urgency may be less. When patients present for same-day surgery (1–4 hours), the focus of the staff is different from the focus in a mental health outpatient facility. Staff education must be planned for the specific needs, practice, and competencies required for patient care, no matter what the setting.

The educator is responsible for teaching the staff to provide patient care in a certain period, whether it be hours, days, or months. Time requirements determine the approach to staff, objectives, content, and evaluation of educational events.

Each major setting in health care involves some knowledge and competency expectations that you are required to help the staff retain. No one expects an educator to be an expert in every medical specialty, but educators are expected to have the ability to plan and be resourceful in meeting educational needs in a wide variety of specialties and settings.

5. Why does it matter whom I am teaching?

The audience that you teach is as diverse as the type of patient—cardiac, diabetic, 2-day old or 82-year-old; trauma victim or person with chronic illness; mentally disturbed or mentally healthy. One of the first skills that you learn as an educator is how to assess the type of people (audience) who will present for instruction. You should know what (content) to teach them and what they already know (see Chapter 12). As you learn instructional design, one of the first steps is to determine who the audience is. You also need to understand why they are present for the learning experience. Teaching the staff to do cardiopulmonary resuscitation (CPR) is quite different from teaching the executive team why it is important to maintain contact with the American Heart Association for CPR information and materials. The approach is different; the content is different; and the level of content, focus, and selection of media are different.

All educators should remember that people do not like to have their time wasted. Teach them something they do not know, and you can link with what they do know. Make the application of gained knowledge immediately apparent.

Many vendors produce programs that educators may consider purchasing. The primary caution is not to use the program as a stand-alone educational event. Purchased programs need to be customized for the audience based on their experience. Vendor-created programs are often quite basic. It is the educator's responsibility to see that the content level of the program meets the audience's needs. Vendor programs need a solid introduction by a facilitator who can connect the program content with the audience's specific needs as well as debrief the audience after the program is completed.

One of the greatest challenges for any instructor is a group that is "required" but does not want to be in attendance. Mandatory education is difficult to plan and deliver. The people who do not want to attend affect others in the audience and distract the instructor.

If you know who is in the audience in advance, you can be prepared to establish a positive environment for learning with opportunities for the learner to be actively involved.

6. Where does the educator fit in the organizational structure? Why is placement an interesting factor?

You may expect a straightforward answer: The department of education should answer to the chief nursing officer. The reality is far from that simple. Each health care facility has good reasons for its design of the function of education. Each facility has a customized organizational structure for the process of educating staff, making the possibilities endless.

Part of the answer to this question is grounded not in the precise placement but in the fact that a great deal of thought and discussion went into the decision. Much of the success of an educational effort depends on the characteristics, qualities, attitudes, and adaptability of the people involved (educators and other leaders). One department of education changed its position in the organization and the person to whom it reported four times in three years—and did so successfully. Why? Because of the adaptability, leadership, and focus of the nurse leading the charge.

7. Distinguish between centralized and decentralized education structure.

In a **centralized structure** of nursing education, all educational efforts of patient care staff are coordinated through one department, and all educators answer to one person, who in turn answers to someone higher in the organizational structure. The advantage of this structure is that efforts can be coordinated more effectively around resources and priorities. The disadvantage is that it is not as close to the patient's bedside, and some needs slip through the crack. In some facilities, this approach is effective. The key is to understand expectations and responsibilities.

A **decentralized structure** can take infinite shapes and designs. Examples include the following:

- Educators are assigned to nursing sections (e.g., medical-surgical, surgical, critical care).
- Educators are assigned to service line leadership; for example, a center for cardiac excellence, which may include a critical care unit, open-heart surgery, medical telemetry, pulmonary unit, cardiac step-down, cardiac catheterization, medical units, respiratory therapy, and perhaps noninvasive vascular labs.
- Educators may be assigned to the service line as one part of their duties and to the department of education for the other part of their duties. In this arrangement, gray areas abound. To whom does the educator ultimately answer, and how is her or his time really divided? A 50–50 time split is rare in real life. This approach can work, but only if the educator is highly flexible and self-directed.

8. To whom should the nurse educator report?

Reporting structure for the educator depends on the facility-wide structure of education. A unit educator may answer directly to the unit manager because the manager created the position from other available staffing hours. In some facilities the educator covers service lines and reports to the service-line director. Other facilities have a department of education that coordinates most or all educational activities in the facility. This department usually reports through the nursing leadership of the hospital. Often the nursing leader responsible for the department of education is someone who has a strong belief in the value of education. It is not unusual for this leader to have other services also.

The "who" is not as important as your relationship with this person. Educators need to understand what is expected of them in the organization and to have information about organizational goals so that the educational goals support these initiatives.

9. My hospital does not seem to value education. What can I do?

In the current health care environment with a shrinking workforce, it is difficult to believe that a hospital would not value education. Medical care changes so fast and technology is exploding in so many areas that hospitals have the responsibility and obligation to keep their staff current. Just as Ghandi believed that an individual citizen makes a difference, so can one nurse in any health care facility. It will not be easy and requires unprecedented commitment, but one person can make a difference. It may not be that the hospital does not value education; it may be that it has not had a leader to help the initiative. Be the leader.

10. What strategies may be helpful in leading an organization to value education?

1. *Gain an ally in your nurse manager.* Work with the nurse manager to improve orientation. Together you can demonstrate that better-oriented and better-prepared new nurses are more productive and more likely to stay employed with the institution.
2. *Many books, articles, and other resources offer information* about orientation, education of staff, and improving care through the educational process. Read everything so that you can be the best educator possible. You might begin by reading the references in this book.
3. *Keep good records and data* about the educational programs that you create and demonstrate to the leadership that the improvements are a result of a focused plan of education.
4. *Place educational events on bulletin boards* for all to see.
5. *Gain allies among your peers.* Choose a few other nurses to help you, and create a plan for inservicing the staff that will meet the needs of the unit or service line. Work with these nurses and the nurse manager to present an educational component at all staff meetings.
6. *Make education fun.* Many books contain games and exercises for learning. Avoid excessive use of lectures. Discussions are great way to involve the staff, and brainstorming sessions can be creative and fun. There should always be a purpose for any game or exercise (even if the purpose is to have fun). Games help break the ice for staff who are not used to organized methods of education.
7. *Get feedback from the remaining staff.* If a new skill or procedure has been taught, follow up in a month to see if the staff is practicing the procedure as taught and how the education helped them learn the skills.
8. *Ask physicians to participate in the educational process.* Concentrate initially on physicians who admit frequently to your unit and can provide feedback about improvements in patient care.
9. As education on your unit begins to show positive results, *conduct a simple needs assessment* (see Chapter 8). Once the assessment is completed, you can establish a 3-month, 6-month, or 1-year plan for your unit. By this time, your unit's dedication to education probably is getting attention from other units and leaders—you can make a difference.
10. *Become informed about the educational expectations* of the Joint Commission for Accreditation of Healthcare Organizations, and be sure your unit meets all of these requirements.
11. *Network with other facilities,* and learn how they approach education on the unit level, service line, support departments, and hospital-wide. Many resources are available for educators; do not try to reinvent the wheel, or you may become frustrated. Many websites can help you, such as the websites for *Training* magazine and most nursing organizations.
12. *Get involved in local nursing organizations* to see what additional resources are available.
13. After you have some experience and feel comfortable in your own knowledge and philosophy of education, *make an appointment to talk with the chief nursing officer*. Have a plan ready in writing that will demonstrate your success and how it affects the organization.

14. Take courses in education at the local college, such as adult learning, curriculum design, program evaluation, and presentation skills. These courses may help you become more knowledgeable in leading the education initiative.

11. What is the major resource needed by educators?

The major resource needed for educators is *time*. For educators on a nursing unit, time is required to plan, prepare, present, and evaluate. Some hospitals and facilities allot a portion of a full-time equivalent for education, and some educators are figured into the staffing pattern on the unit.

- When educators are full-time employees and assigned to specific units, they need time with the staff—in other words, time to educate.
- Hospitals are highly conscious of paying overtime for staff; this can affect time allotted for staff education.
- If the time allotted to education is about 30 minutes in staff meetings, it simply is not enough to keep staff abreast of the changes in medical care.
- Educators need to establish educational programs that fit the time allocated as well as meet the needs of the staff and unit. Use your time well. Use their time efficiently.
- Budgeted dollars for education are necessary. Most educators have lived on slim budgets, but it helps if some dollars are allocated for the resources included in questions 12 and 13. Most managers dedicated to education are quite creative in finding financial support for education within their budgets. Don't be afraid to state your needs.

12. List the resources that are essential to educators.

- Space to work in. Educators need an office or cubicle in which to organize the process of education and keep records and other resources.
- Educators must have a computer dedicated to their work and available to them as needed. It is ideal if the computer has e-mail, word-processing software, spreadsheet software, and a graphics package. A presentation graphics package such as Power Point makes creating visual aids much easier. Get connected to the Internet. It is a fabulous resource for research, education, and clinical care.
- Reference books and journals about education/staff development, orientations, specialty area (e.g., cardiovascular care, long-term care), games, and exercises are needed to enhance the learning process. Some hospitals have adequate libraries that include nursing resources. Use it!

13. What additional resources are particularly helpful?

- As an educator, you need to stay up to date. It is helpful if you can attend regional or national meetings in your specialty or in the area of education. Join nursing organizations such as American Association of Critical Care Nurses (AACN), Oncology Nursing Society, or the Association of Operating Room Nurses. Networking at these meetings can be invaluable.
- A classroom is a great resource—a place close to your unit or department that is dedicated to use by educators. Although most hospitals have a shortage of rooms for education, a conference room or classroom can be a time-saving and handy resource.
- Keep a supply of toys on the table for attendees. Adults like to have something in their hands while sitting in education sessions. Go to toy stores, grocery stores, office supply stores, and specialty shops. Suggestions include Koosh balls, stick figures, wands with glitter inside, and puzzles. Hint: stay away from toys that make sounds.
- Supplies of all types, including colorful computer paper, seasonal paper (e.g., Christmas, Halloween, Valentine's Day) for eye-catching announcements on bulletin boards, and basic tools such as markers, masking tape, easel markers that do not bleed through, and colorful pens. Visit your local office supply store or locate a teachers' store near you

14. Who should do the teaching?

There may be a simple answer to this question. One of the greatest assets of any organization is the human asset. Health care facilitates are no exception. Every hospital, clinic, long-term care facility, or outpatient facility has great human potential. Educators need to identify who has the talent to do the job and then draft, persuade, and convince that person to become involved in the educational process.

Whether the setting is a small facility, clinic, or large teaching hospital, the person assigned to responsibility and accountability for planning, implementing, and evaluating education should *want* to do the job. Managers who randomly select the best patient care nurse for promotion to educator, without consideration of the nurse's desire to teach, may be creating a future disaster. New learners know when the teacher wants to be teaching them, and adult learners learn best from caring and compassionate educators who have learned the skills of coaching and mentoring. Choose your educator(s) carefully. It is better to develop a nurse or other health care professional who has never been an educator than to push someone, no matter how good his or her skills, into teaching. Everyone pays the price. Set the educator up for success, and the manager succeeds too.

When you are looking for help in a program, the person doing the teaching should be the expert. But not all experts want to teach, nor do they have the skills to teach others. This is where the educator can be a great resource to the content expert. The educator can teach the expert the necessary skills found throughout this book, such as how to assess needs, prepare instruction, and optimize presentation. The educator is responsible for ensuring that guest speakers (experts) are set up to succeed.

If the educator is the expert, perhaps the educator should deliver the content. Educators who are dedicated to a unit or service line may conduct most of the educational sessions, but it is always good to know teaching resources within the hospital. If you need a class about assessing patients with head injury, go to the neurosurgery unit and find a good nurse or a physician to teach it. Depending on the content, you may consider offering a variety of teachers. Too many educators try to carry the load alone when it is unnecessary. Build a list of who can teach what, and use it to broaden the educational experience for the learner.

Depending on "visiting experts" can be a frustrating part of your job if the expert is late in giving you the objectives, outlines, and handouts. Ask each visiting expert to complete an instructor's workplan (see below), keep it on file for reference, and have it available for later presentations by the same person.

Instructional Workplan

Class topic:
Presenter's name:
Date and time for presentation:
A. Target audience:

B. Objectives:
 1.
 2.
 3.
C. Content outline:

D. Teaching methods *(circle all that apply)*:

1. Lecture	3. Role-play	5. Group discussion
2. Interactive exercises	4. Audiovisual	6. Demonstration

E. Visual equipment needs

1. Flip chart	3. Overhead projector	5. Other:
2. VCR	4. Slide projector	

F. Evaluation methods:

Sample instructional workplan. (© BJ Crim, AW Hood, Partners in Learning, Dallas, TX; used with permission.)

15. When should I use quality assurance (QA) data?

Educators need to know not only how to collect data but also when to use it. Many "data" are presented to staff. The educator should clearly relate QA data to the purpose of the educational session, change in practice, or new protocol.

QA data should be used to identify patient care gaps, and educational strategies should be developed to fill this gap. For example, if your unit is tracking an indicator of how well the patient's pain is controlled and the data show an opportunity for improvement, use the data to show the need for a review or education session; then present the information to the staff in a positive and challenging way.

QA data can be helpful in providing needed knowledge to staff. If patients on your unit have a higher postoperative infection rate than patients on other units and the quality team has identified the reasons, use the data to teach the staff how to improve the infection rate and get them involved in tracking the infection rate.

Educators should watch the QA data for instances when improvements in the data are a direct (or perhaps somewhat indirect) outcome of education. Helping the staff and management see the relationship of education to indicator improvement is essential. This strategy proves why education can make a difference in patient care and the bottom line of the facility. Keep good records.

To be more knowledgeable about data that they use, educators should understand the concepts, principles, and data-gathering methods found in continuous quality improvement, total quality management, and process improvement theories. This information is available in most public as well as medical libraries. The leaders in the field are Joseph Juran, W.E. Deming, and Phillip Crosby.

16. How can the gap between education and clinical nursing be bridged?

This question probably is one of the most important issues related to education. Health care facilities, as discussed earlier, have many different organizational structures. Education is a vital part of keeping staff current in their practice, but the patient care units are also vital and have special needs and wants. How do we create a smooth, collaborative, and efficient way of working together?

The first questions that need answering are obvious: "Is there is a gap between education and clinical nursing in the organization? If so, why?"

The most important aspect of preventing or bridging a gap is to have good working relationships. Covey discusses in depth the issue of building relationships in *Seven Habits of Highly Effective People*.[2] The author recommends that every educator read this book. We have relationships with our spouse, children, friends, and colleagues. Relationships do not just happen; they takes time, effort, and work to build and maintain. Educators should establish a plan to build a good working relationship with the manager and staff of the units with which they work and then to maintain these relationships. If you are a new educator or have been assigned a new nursing unit, spend time finding out what their special educational and development needs are, and obtain this information from everyone involved (see Chapter 8). Spend time talking with the staff, observing their work, and discussing issues with them. Educators first need to gain the staffs' trust and communicate a positive interest in their success. Most gaps in relationship can be tracked to a breakdown in communication; it is best to dedicate time to keeping the lines of communication open.

Adults like to be involved in planning programs that affect their job. Get them involved by having them serve on planning committees, completing surveys, and even teaching some of the classes. When you observe a skills or practice need, ask for staff input. Take care to spread participation throughout all staff; do not stick with the same staff all of the time. From the perspective of the staff, there is a fine line between overusing willing people and dumping on them. Consider using the staff who do not always agree with you; getting them actively involved in improving patient care can change behaviors. You may be surprised to find them strong supporters in future projects.

Another important aspect of maintaining relationships is to be vigilant in your follow-up with the staff concerning programs, inservices, or any educator responsibility. As stated in the preplanning of an event, touch base with the staff on the content, speakers, and other elements of the planning. For instance, if you are planning an internship or orientation for new staff, talk to the existing staff about what should be included, what has worked and what has not, and what would improve the experience of the new person on their unit. During the program, ask all participants, "How are things going?" Do not wait until the orientation is over to find out that it did not go well or that something could have been changed to make it better. When the internship or event is over, ask for staff input on possible improvements. Thus, the educator must be in touch with staff (1) during preplanning, (2) as the program is progressing, and (3) at the end of the program. Demonstrate to the staff your appreciation for their time and commitment to ensuring a good outcome. They will learn from you and you from them. A positive outcome will be that you are highly visible and interactive with the staff; they will respect these qualities in you.

When an educator is planning an educational event that represents the nursing unit or practice, they should ensure that the content matches reality. In other words, provide learners with knowledge and skills that they can use on the unit. One of the biggest gaps between education and clinical practice is that patient care providers feel that what is being taught is not what they really do. This is a fine line to walk, because what is "done" may not be how it "should" be done. If the educator has done a good job of building relationships with the staff, the difference is not so difficult to correct; but if there is a lack of trust or a gap between the two, a major conflict may develop. Be sure that, before you add a new practice or skill to a program for new nurses, you have introduced it to the existing staff. Use as your motto "Set everyone up for success"—and that includes yourself.

17. How do you measure whether you are visible enough and sufficiently engaged with the staff?

Ask yourself the following questions:

- Do I know what is really happening on the unit?
- Am I making changes in what I teach based on my personal observations?
- Am I aware of the issues facing the staff on the unit?
- Are new people succeeding on this unit? Why or why not?

Some staff may feel that the educator is never visible enough, but if you can answer the above questions, you are probably meeting the expectations as an educator for the unit. In order to bridge the gap between education and nursing practice, you need the support of management—all the way up in the organization. Management support means that you share a common philosophy for the expectations and desired outcomes of education. Obtain support for what you feel needs to be done for the units. The relationship with the specific unit manager is vital to this goal because he or she can make things happen for the educator. Work at building a collaborative relationship with management. The simple answer to gap questions is to work at the relationships and reap the rewards.

18. How do I plan my own development?

Every educator needs to have a personal short- and long-term development plan for his or her professional growth. There are many ways to approach your development as an educator. First, put it in writing for yourself and your manager. The following issues should be considered:

1. Look at the job expectations and your knowledge base. If you see areas in which you need more knowledge, get it. For example, your job may require you to be an instructor in advanced cardiac life support. You may need to plan a review of the content of the program, work in the critical care unit once in a while, and observe a course. Once you identify what you need, create a plan that meets the need.

2. Attend specialty organization meetings to learn what the issues are and whether you need to learn more about the topic. Find a way to do this.

3. Take classes toward an advanced degree at a local college or through a distance learning program.

4. Read all of the time. Read journals and books, or go on-line to find information that you need.

5. Set short-term and long-term goals for yourself. Keep a log of how you are doing, and review it at least monthly. Keep your manager informed of your progress.

6. Find a mentor. He or she may be a member of your organization or someone across the country. Mentors are great resources for the developing educator.

7. Step outside the box of clinical issues, and develop a plan to learn more about the job of the educator. Examples include adult learning principles, curriculum design, public speaking, budget development, and writing skills.

8. Educators should support life-long learning. Be a role model to others.

9. Start by reading this book—from cover to cover.

BIBLIOGRAPHY

1. Bell CR: Managers as Mentors. San Francisco, Berrett-Koehler, 1996.
2. Covey SR: The Seven Habits of Highly Effective People. New York, Simon & Schuster, 1989.
3. Daloz LA: Effective Teaching and Mentoring. San Francisco, Jossey-Bass, 1986.
4. Galbraith MW (ed): Adult Learning Methods. Malabar, FL, Krieger, 1990.
5. Galbraith MW (ed): Facilitating Adult Learning: A Transactional Process. Malabar, FL, Krieger, 1991.
6. Knowles MS: The Making of an Adult Educator. San Francisco, Jossey-Bass, 1989.
7. Leebov W, Scott, G: Health Care Managers in Transition. San Francisco, Jossey-Bass, 1990.
8. Merriam SB, Cunningham PM (eds): Handbook of Adult and Continuing Education. San Francisco, Jossey-Bass, 1989.
9. Newstrom JW, Scannell EE: Games Trainers Play. New York, McGraw-Hill, 1980.
10. Newstrom JW, Scannell, EE: Still More Games Trainers Play. New York, McGraw-Hill, 1980.
11. Queeney DS: Assessing Needs in Continuing Education. San Francisco, Jossey-Bass, 1995.

4. EDUCATOR COMPETENCIES

Angela C. Wolff, MSN, RN

1. What is the difference between educator competence and competencies?

In education and other allied health professions, the concept of competence has been studied extensively, and variations of competence have been identified as either a product or a process. For the purpose of this chapter, *competence* is viewed as process-oriented, implying that competence is developed and manifested as a process over time and with experience. As such, the development of competence may occur in stages or as a trajectory from novice to expert. Motivation, interest, energy, and commitment are required to help you deal with the factors that influence your competence. Because competence is not seen as a constant state, your feelings may fluctuate between anxiety and tension, comfort, and a sense of empowerment.

Competencies are specific performance statements that originate from experience, observation, and validation. These statements need to be based on the actual clinical activities and responsibilities performed by competent educators. In addition, competencies should be considerate of situational and contextual factors. For example, if you were a neophyte versus an experienced educator, you would most likely demonstrate competencies at a different level that should be evaluated accordingly.

2. What knowledge, skills, and attitudes do I need as an educator?

To be successful as an educator, you need to possess leadership, management, and communication skills; clinical expertise; and political savvy.[6] The competencies that you require can be categorized in the cognitive, psychomotor, and affective/attitudinal domains.

Cognitive domain

- Applies nursing knowledge (e.g., theoretical, personal, practical) and organizational philosophies.
- Demonstrates the educational process (e.g., principles of adult learning and the learning paradigm, program development, educational philosophies, needs assessment).
- Critical thinking skills, including the ability to solve problems and make clinical and teacher judgments.

Psychomotor domain

- Clinical skills
- Teaching skills
- Expert learner skills
- Physical and motor skills

Affective domain

- Interpersonal skills (e.g., verbal, written, and computer)
- Political savvy (e.g., "reading" the work environment, building credibility, helping the supervisor succeed)
- Ability to reflect critically about your personal characteristics.
- Attitudes (e.g., enjoyment of nursing), values, and beliefs that complement nursing and teaching roles.
- Professional behaviors (e.g., role model, responsibility for actions, lifelong learner).

Specific competencies required of novice nurse educators are further delineated by the National Nursing Staff Development Organization.[8] Identified are six core standards and competence statements for administration, human resources, material resources and facilities, educational design, records and reports, and professional practice.

3. What is the relationship between confidence and competence?

To be competent, you need to develop a sense of confidence that you can succeed as a clinician and a teacher. This confidence in your ability to be successful is also called self-efficacy. Educators with more self-confidence feel a greater sense of control over their environment. Self-confidence is necessary for the evolving process of competence; the two concepts have a reciprocal interdependent relationship. When you view yourself as successful and competent, your self-confidence is enhanced. Feelings of pride and respect heighten your self-confidence; the more self-confidence developed, the easier it is to engage in self-learning activities directed towards enhancing your competence. It is reasonable to speculate that your ability and perceived self-confidence, as a clinician and as a teacher, have a strong influence on your competence as an educator.

4. Describe the leadership skills on which I should focus to become a successful educator.

One role of an educator is change agent. As such, you should possess strong leadership, management, and communication skills. Political savvy is also an asset for implementing changes in practice, introducing an innovation, or advocating for student-centered learning.[6] This role frequently involves leadership activities such as chairing working groups, conducting meetings, monitoring staff progress, and advocating for clinical practice. Leadership abilities include providing feedback, being assertive, making decisions, analyzing problems, building a work team, negotiating, delegating, facilitating, resolving conflict, developing programs, managing a budget, taking initiative, and dealing with system-level changes. As a leader, you must also be able to reconcile the differing and present needs of staff while meeting the present and future needs of the organization as a whole.

5. What interpersonal skills are necessary for the job of educator?

Excellent interpersonal skills are vital for educators. The staff with whom you work often determine your capability by assessing your written and verbal skills. Verbal interpersonal skills required of educators include assertiveness, listening, empathy, problem-analysis, negotiation, and conflict resolution. Such skills are often used during consultations with and presentations for staff. Written communication skills are reflected in memos, letters, e-mail, educational flyers, and educational materials. In addition, it is extremely important that you "walk the talk" in role-modeling behaviors that you expect of your learners.

Educators are expected to react with confidence to unanticipated statements and unexpected educational activities with an effective problem-solving response (e.g., on-the-spot learning situations and negative reactions from learners). Furthermore, interpersonal skills are required to assess the needs of learners, evaluate the learning situation, and advocate for quality education programs for nurses. Effective computer and written skills are essential for all aspects of an educator's role, including program development, strategic planning, and proposal writing.

6. Do I need three years of clinical experience before I can apply for a staff development educator role?

There are two perspectives about clinical expertise and educational expertise. First, the person is an educational expert, rather than a clinical expert, who facilitates the learning process. Second, the educator is a clinical expert with supplementary educational expertise. In addition to these perspectives is the common assumption that a competent nurse will be a competent clinical educator. However, this is not always the reality.

Several authors have stated that nursing practice is a necessary requirement for being able to teach in the clinical setting; however, empirical evidence in the nursing literature fails to substantiate this claim. When you make the transition from clinical practitioner to educator, you may notice that you tend to rely on your abilities as a clinician. In this instance, your experience (e.g., nursing practice, teaching, formal education) provides a venue for you to acquire, integrate, and apply the knowledge, skills, and attitudes necessary for developing competence in your new role. Yet measuring experience in terms of actual time spent in practice is insufficient for identifying your competence as an educator.[1,7,14] Rather, the development of your competence as a clinical educator is continual; it is based on your cognitive ability to learn and gain meaning from your experiences. In other words, experience is acquired when preconceived ideas and actions are challenged, refined, or rejected. Thus, gaining meaning from experiences is achieved through critical thinking, problem-solving, reflection, and self-awareness.[11]

Although some people have assumed that the passing of time is necessary for competence to develop, some aspects of competence may, in fact, deteriorate with experience. For example, as the skills of an individual's role become more rote and less lively, he or she may continue to use the same skills. For experience to have an effect on clinical teaching practice, it must reflect continuous professional development (e.g., gaining meaning from an event or situation) rather than the completion of a series of repeated activities over time.[3]

In short, clinical experience is one factor that may facilitate your transition to the educator role, boost your self-confidence, and influence others' perceptions of your credibility. However, the debate of "how much" and "what type" of nursing practice remains unanswered or is perhaps best determined by you, the learner. To learn and grow, teachers also must have an attitude of inquiry, a willingness to improve, an ability to gain insight, and a commitment to lifelong learning. To develop and maintain your competence as an educator, you must assume responsibility to continue to develop personally and professionally. An important predictor of your success as an educator is your ability to gain meaning from personal experiences and, if necessary, to modify your behavior accordingly.[15]

7. What factors may enhance or hinder my development as a competent educator?

The process of competence is situation-specific and context-bound. Your ability to deal with your surroundings is influenced by personal (internal) factors and environmental (external) factors that affect the course and outcome of the process of developing competence.

Internal factors include nursing practice; knowledge related to teaching and learning; personal qualities; communication abilities; and self perceptions, beliefs, values, and expectations.

External factors include support and/or mentoring; familiarity with clinical agencies; orientation to the role; stable work environment; organizational systems; health reform; role description; and perceived credibility.

Receiving support is necessary to facilitate your transition through the competence process. Educators receiving support feel empowered, self-confident, and less anxious. Because anxiety is negatively correlated with competence, it is paramount for you, as an educator, to find the support you need in this new role. Further consequences of support have been identified as perceived control, positive affect, sense of stability, and recognition of self-worth. Overall, these positive feelings contribute to job satisfaction and ambition to further your development as a competent educator.

8. As an educator, should I continue to be directly involved with clinical practice?

Involvement in activities in the clinical unit and organization is an effective way to gain visibility and to keep abreast of clinical issues that may need addressing. You may chose to maintain your clinical expertise by setting aside one to two days as "clinical days," making frequent clinical rounds, or assisting during times of high workload. The purpose of the clinical days, for example, may be to mentor a new nursing employee, to allow staff to observe you in the educator role from a clinical perspective, or to build and maintain your credibility. Moreover, working directly with staff and providing direct patient care can provide teachable moments and an opportunity to reinforce and evaluate previous learning sessions. Spending time with direct patient care communicates to staff the importance of education in informing and contributing to clinical practice. To maintain visibility you may also want to involve staff in your projects as an educator. This approach may encourage staff to "buy into" a particular educational program.

9. What are common role descriptions and performance expectations of educators?

Most clinical educators are responsible for clinical and professional development of staff (e.g., orientation, educational programming, evaluation of staff competency). However, you also may be asked to perform a combined role as staff educator, patient educator, and unit manager. This combination is a challenging and perhaps unrealistic expectation, because staff development can be a full-time responsibility. To provide quality educational programs, time must be dedicated to their development and delivery.

In the United States, the National Nursing Staff Development Organization[8] identifies competency statements and critical behaviors expected of nursing clinical educators. In Canada, the

Registered Nurses Association of British Columbia[10] provides standards and indicators for nurse educators in that province. Additional authors, such as Lane,[4] Marciniak,[5] and Naughton and Strobel,[9] also outline various performance expectations for nurse educators. Generally speaking, your responsibilities include educator (e.g., orientation, ongoing staff education), researcher (e.g., collaboration on development of standards, policies, procedures, and nursing quality improvement programs; using and conducting research), and consultant for clinical and administrative issues.[12] You also are expected to keep current with educational trends such as focus on the learning (i.e., process-oriented) paradigm vs. the instructional (i.e., product-oriented) paradigm.

10. Describe the process for evolving from a novice and to an expert educator.

Most basic nursing programs do not include concepts of the educational process in their curricula. Thus, your transition from the role of expert nurse clinician to staff development educator may be turbulent and anxiety-provoking. Attaining competence as a clinical educator entails a three-phased maturation process that is contextual and situation-specific[15]:

1. The first phase, dealing with self-learning needs, is a **period of adjustment** in which neophyte clinical educators confront the difficulties associated with making the transition to the clinical teacher role. This phase is characterized by uncertainty and lack of confidence. Aside from the usual anxieties associated with a new role, many neophyte clinical teachers are overwhelmed with the perception that they need to "know everything" and are worried about not being viewed as "credible" by their colleagues. Educators in this phase bring clinical expertise but often have limited educational skills and practical teaching experience. Many educators begin teaching by emulating teaching behaviors that they observed as students. In this phase of developing competence, educators need to focus on self-learning needs before focusing on the needs of the learner.

2. At the beginning of the second phase, clinical educators feel more self-confident and comfortable in their role. They concentrate on **developing a unique teaching style** by challenging old assumptions about teaching and learning and discovering new alternatives. Through a process of trial and error, educators test, revise, and refine their unique teaching style. In addition to reading, observing, and conferring with other clinical educators, they adopt other activities to learn how to teach: feedback, evaluation, and reflection. By focusing on student-centered learning, educators continue to refine their teaching style by developing a greater appreciation for students as individuals with unique learning needs and challenges. In this phase, educators become more skilled at matching their teaching style with the learners' needs. They also became competent in giving feedback and evaluating learners.

3. During the third phase, clinical educators develop a greater appreciation for and understanding of how to integrate their abilities as a clinical educator within the **broader context of nursing education**. Educators in this phase are perceptive and skilled. They are risk takers, have intuitive grasp of each learning situation, are committed to nursing education, and appreciate the complexities involved in fostering learning. They use role-modeling as a predominant teaching method and encourage multiple ways of learning while considering the learners' styles and needs.

Key Descriptors of the Three Phases of the Competence Process

PHASE 1	PHASE 2	PHASE 3
Concrete	Concrete to abstract	Highly abstract
Self-centered	Self-centered to collegial	Autonomous
Surviving	Task-oriented/mechanistic	Flexible
Rigid	Unstable to empirical	Adaptable
Fearful	Testing to expending	Synthetical
	Basic conceptualist	Highly conceptual
	Emerging reflection	Analytical
	Conformity crisis	Actualized

From Lane AJ: Developing healthcare educators: The application of a conceptual model. J Nurs Staff Devel 12:252–259, 1996, with permission.

11. What type of orientation program is appropriate for educators?

Each nurse comes to the staff development educator role at a different level. Therefore, methods used for orienting an experienced educator are not necessarily the same as those required for a neophyte educator. Your orientation and ongoing professional development are paramount to role assimilation and development. Orientation programs provide a means by which you, as a new educator, are introduced to the philosophy, goals, policies, procedures, role expectations, physical facilities, and competencies pertaining to educators. The National Nursing Staff Development Organization[8] provides competency statements, critical behaviors, learning resources, and evaluation methods to assist in planning orientation programs for nurses who are new to the educator role.

Look for orientation programs that are comprehensive and may include the following components: (1) descriptions of the educator's roles, responsibilities, and competencies; (2) opportunities to plan, develop, and direct educational programs; and (3) information about organizing and maintaining competency profiles and records.[4,5,9,13] You also want to have an orientation program that is flexible in meeting specific needs and leveled according to your expertise as a clinical educator. It should allow you to choose learning activities that match your learning style.

An effective and well-rounded orientation program should provide opportunities for self-assessment such as identifying capabilities and determining strengths and weaknesses. After completion of the self-assessment, a mutually designed learning plan should be developed. This plan should include planned activities, set time lines, and evaluation methods for your professional development in the identified areas. The program should extend over 3–6 months, during which you can implement the learning plan, receive feedback, and self-evaluate. The plan should be reassessed and revised as needed. Finally, a summative and formative evaluation of the developmental plan should be done. Appropriate feedback may be included on your performance evaluation. Some programs incorporate the use of mentors or preceptors as a beneficial source of support.[4,5,9,13] (Appendix A contains a sample orientation checklist; Appendix B, a sample competency form.)

12. Are certain personality styles more suited for the educator role?

Personal qualities that facilitate the process of developing competence as an educator include outgoing personality, sense of humor, willingness to learn and to change, personal desire to succeed, acceptance of self, ability to gain insight into personal behaviors, natural ability to reflect, ability to challenge oneself, attitude of commitment, spirit of inquiry, and integrity. Educators displaying a variety of these personal qualities often have greater feelings of self-confidence and competence.[15] Many teachers find that a quest for knowledge is an important component of becoming competent and avoiding complacency. To keep up to date, you need to possess sensitivity and responsiveness, feel secure with change, and seek out opportunities to continue to develop holistically.[5]

13. As an educator, what methods can I use to organize my work?

At times you may be overwhelmed with the scope of responsibility of the role. Teamwork, collegial collaboration, and alliance building are essential to achieving your work goals. Moreover, a helpful way of organizing your responsibilities is to determine their importance and urgency. An activity is deemed important if you or the organization find it valuable (i.e., the activity contributes to the mission and role requirements and is a high priority). An activity is urgent if you or others in the organization think that it requires immediate attention. The best use of your time requires you to focus activities that emphasize importance versus urgency. Therefore, allocate time to those events that are (1) important and urgent (e.g., crises, pressing problems, project deadlines, meetings) or (2) important and not urgent (e.g., preparation and planning, relationships building, prevention).[2] Avoid spending time on unimportant urgent or nonurgent matters (e.g., interruptions, trivia busywork, time wasters, irrelevant mail). Others components of keeping organized are to allow "white space" for desk time in your calendar, to maximize your in-house resources (e.g., administration staff, library), and to delegate.

14. How can educators become more proficient with computers?

Increasingly you will be required to use computers for both external and internal communication (see Chapter 16). If you have limited computer skills, the best way to learn is to practice. As with anything new, learn by the method that best matches your learning style. If you learn by visual or auditory methods, you may decide that a computer course best suits your need. If you are a hands-on learner, spend time exploring your computer programs. Most computer programs incorporate a pop-up function that defines the function of each button. For example, if you pass the mouse over the symbol that looks like a printer, a window will appear saying "print." Most computer programs also have a built-in help feature that allows you to ask questions or perform a search by topic. Also consider using other available internal resources, such as the information systems department and administrative support staff.

15. Why is customer service important to educators?

As previously stated, most educators are responsible for clinical and professional development of nursing staff within their organization; hence, the nursing staff is the customer. The climate of the workplace is critical to the kind of product, or learning outcome. Education that is based on a need identified by you or your organization is not likely to succeed because the learners need to be active participants in all aspects of the education process. It is important to provide good customer service by meeting the adult learning needs through learner-centered education. Adults learn best when the content is life-focused, meets a specific need, enhances their self-concept, and builds on previous life experiences. If you are hoping to change behavior, provide knowledge, or teach a skill, you need to focus on the learners' needs. When learners feel supported in their environment, it creates positive physiologic effects in their brain such as improved memory, verbal functioning, flexible thinking, creative problem-solving, and social interactions. In short, without good customer service, learning may not occur.

Appendix A

Center for Education and Staff Development Orientation Checklist

Name: ______________________ Position: ________________ Start Date________________

TOPIC/SKILL	REVIEWED BY	DATE
General Information		
Tour of department		
Introduction to CESD staff		
Introduction to human resources staff		
Assign desk, get keys		
Ensure ergonomic setup of desk, chair, computer		
Discuss shelves, equipment, work area layout		
Restrooms		
Staff phone numbers		
Hospital map		
Orient to department routine • Breaks • Lunch • Mail/mailboxes • Distribution.routing		
Customer service • First one here opens all doors, turns on copier, printer • Last one to leave turns everything off, checks doors are locked		

Continued on following page

TOPIC/SKILL	REVIEWED BY	DATE
Customer service *(cont.)* • Covering phones when secretary off—voice mail access numbers • Sign to use when everyone out of the department		
Time cards/paychecks		
Mileage reimbursement		
Telephones • Transfers/hold • How to answer • Voice mail • Intercom • Phone book		
Telephone list, useful phone numbers		
Order business cards		
Order appointment book and other desk supplies		
Draft announcement of position		
Safety • Location of exits, extinguishers • Role in fire, disaster • Safety manuals		
Department-specific Items		
Review of department mission, vision, philosophy, goals, organizational charts		
Meet with each department member to review their responsibilities • • • •		
Meet with division leader		
Meet with education secretary to review: • Registration book • Label lists • "It's Friday" submissions • Quarterly calendar • Purchase orders • Food orders • Supply requests • Copy requests • Video library list • Self-learning pkts and masters • Mandatory posters • Equipment/tape sign out • Program attendance data entry • Petty cash/record book/receipts • Department keys (storage room, bayfront class, etc.)		
Tour of tape/equipment storage areas		
Review CESD policies/guidelines		
Review nursing contact hour process		

Continued on following page

TOPIC/SKILL	REVIEWED BY	DATE
Review safety/RTK materials • Codes • Location of exits, extinguishers • Roles in a disaster • Call list • Department hazards		
Review QI plan for department		
Arranging teleconferences/video conferences		
Arranging audio conferences		
Arranging televideo Process for recordkeeping/files		
Equipment orientation • Overheads • Slide projector • Copier • Fax • Easels • Computer • Laser printer • Color printer • Shredder • TV/VCR • Laptop • LCD projector • Speaker • Audio conferencing equipment		
Individual Position		
Program planning • Needs assessment • Content • Outline/objectives • Contacting speakers • Handouts • Advertising		
Program implementation • Sign-ins • Introductions • Develop evaluation form		
Program evaluation • Summary • Measuring effectiveness • Revise as needed		
Productivity reports: what to record, how to record		
Journal subscriptions		
Staff development competencies		
Computer orientation • Windows • MS Word • Share drive, how to find materials • Access/Excel • Calendar Creator		

Continued on following page

TOPIC/SKILL	REVIEWED BY	DATE
Computer orientation *(cont.)* • PowerPoint • Graphics, clipart • E-mail scheduling of rooms, personal schedule, naming surrogates		
Liaison responsibilities		
Committee responsibilities		
Action plan development		
Job description/performance		
Evaluations		
Meet with liaisons:		
Schedule of classes/courses/ activities to observe		
Seminars to attend		
Resources—books to review, orientation manual, literature searches, hospital library, department library		

Comments: ____

____

____

____

Date checklist/orientation competed: ________________
Employee signature: ____________________________

From Hamot Hospital, Erie, PA, with permission.

Appendix B

Center for Education and Staff Development
Staff Development Competency Validation Form

Name: ________________________________ Title: ____________________
Department: ____________________ Start Date: __________ Date Completed __________

Coordinates Educational Opportunities

CRITERIA	METHOD OF MEASURE	VALIDATOR
1. Develops a program idea	Collaborates with liaisons to assess staff needs, current literature, QI data, career development, personal and organizational issues used in program	
2. Plans program to meet identified needs	Content outline, objectives, qualified speakers, principles of adult learning used in program, individualized learning, program promotion	
3. Creates audiovisual aids that are easily understood and project well	Overheads, slides, handouts, etc.	

Continued on following page

Coordinates Educational Opportunities *(Continued)*

CRITERIA	METHOD OF MEASURE	VALIDATOR
4. Coordinates the program so that it runs smoothly	Registrations, sign-in sheet, passes out material, develops evaluation, etc.	
5. Evaluates program	Reviews/uses completed evaluations, measures effectiveness of program, identifies impact, projects future topics, speaker feedback	

Teaching Ability

CRITERIA	METHOD OF MEASURE	VALIDATOR
1. Utilizes adult learning principles in program development/teaching	Describes principles and techniques of adult learning, lists examples of each used appropriately	
2. Communicates program content clearly	Comments on evaluation forms; direct observation, content clearly communicated; intent of program achieved	
3. Utilizes a variety of teaching methods, matches learning method with content and learning style	Content outline lists method, evaluation of teaching method on evaluation forms	
4. Provides feedback to participants	Describes positive and negative reinforcement wand, when to use, comments on evaluation forms	
5. Utilizes group process skills	Learning groups interactive and goal-oriented, describes roles within a group, secures win-win agreements, negotiates	
6. Promotes and uses intellectual versatility, acts as an educational consultant	Demonstrates exploration of broad range of ideas and practices, is creative, uses brainstorming, tree diagrams, etc.	

Validator Signature: ______________________ Employee Signature: ______________________
Supervisor Signature: ____________________
Comments: ____
____
____
____

From Hamot Hospital, Erie, PA, with permission.

BIBLIOGRAPHY

1. Benner P: From Novice to Expert. Menlo Park, CA, Addison-Wesley, 1984.
2. Covey SR: The Seven Habits of Highly Effective People. New York, Simon & Schuster, 1989.
3. Gee K: Competency through being: The enemy within? Br J Nurs 4:637–640, 1995.
4. Lane AJ: Developing healthcare educators: The application of a conceptual model. J Nurs Staff Devel 12: 252–259, 1996.
5. Marciniak CJ: A systematic plan for nurse educator development. J Nurs Staff Devel 13:99–108, 1997.
6. Mateo M, Fahje CJ: The nurse educator role in the clinical setting. J Nurs Staff Devel 14:169–175, 1998.
7. Maynard CA: Relationship of critical thinking ability to professional nursing competence. J Nurs Educ 35:12–18, 1996.
8. National Nursing Staff Development Organization: Guidelines for an Orientation Program for Novice Nursing Professional Development Educators. Pensacola, FL, National Nursing Staff Development Organization, 1994.

9. Naughton DR, Strobel, LM: Assessment of new nurse educators. J Contin Educ Nurs 2:8–11, 1996.
10. Registered Nurses Association of British Columbia: Standards for Nursing Practice in British Columbia. Vancouver, BC, Registered Nurses Association of British Columbia, 2000.
11. Saylor CR: Reflection and professional education: Art, science, and competency. Nurse Educ 15:8–11, 1990.
12. Tutuska AM, Nahigian E: Competency based evaluation: One hospital's approach. J Nurs Staff Devel 13:44–46, 1997.
13. Vezina M, et al: Competency-based orientation for clinical nurse educators. J Nurs Staff Devel 12:311–313, 1996.
14. Watson SJ: An analysis of the concept of experience. J Adv Nurs 16:1117–1121, 1991.
15. Wolff AC: The Process of Maturing as a Competent Clinical Teacher [unpublished master's thesis]. University of British Columbia, Vancouver, BC, 1998.

5. COMPUTER SKILLS FOR EDUCATORS

Kenneth R. *Bowman*, RN, MS

1. Are computer skills really necessary for the staff development educator?

Absolutely. Computer skills are essential. The range of computer skills needed by educators extends from the basics of the personal computer (PC), word processor, and Internet to an understanding of how servers and network systems work in the world of education.

2. How much information about computers does the beginning educator need to get started?

The basics are enough, but the definition of basics depends on what resources are available at your work place. Many hospitals or nursing homes are only beginning to convert to computerization. If your facility does not have the capability to use computerized programs as part of your education process, your focus should be on the PC and word processor. If you happen to be at a facility where computer-based presentations are the norm, you have a much larger job ahead of you.

3. Where should the beginning educator start?

All educators, no matter what type of facility they work in, should start with an understanding of the PC and word-processing. The level of understanding of PCs needed by educators should be higher than that of the average person, but you don't need to be an expert. If you have no hands-on experience with a PC, start by looking for a course in the basics. Courses often are found at local community colleges or technical schools. Start with the type of course directed toward the general public and people about to purchase their first computer. Courses at this level usually include information about processors, random access memory (RAM), and hard drives. Make sure that you are not signing up for a course in how to repair computers; such courses may be labeled PC basics. Basic knowledge of PCs is essential to the educator for such tasks as justifying PCs as budget items for the education department or buying new software. Understanding PCs helps you make better choices in equipment and prevents you from ending up with "leftovers" (someone's retired PC).

4. I know how to use a PC. What's next?

Buying the necessary software is the next step in this process. The most common types of software loaded on PCs are used for typing and business functions. These programs are better known as word processors, spreadsheets, and presentation software. Several packages on the market include this type of software (e.g., Microsoft Office, Lotus Suite). They include a word processor, spreadsheet, and graphics presentation program as part of the package, but they also may include additional items, depending on level. It is important to check the level of the package that you buy. Buying a cheaper package designed for home use may not provide you with the functions that you need as an educator. You may face the expense of buying another copy of software if you are not careful.

Another important point is to make sure that the version of the program is compatible with the software used by other people in your institution and with the operating system. The word *version* is used to refer to changes in software. As software is updated and improved, the version changes. For example, Microsoft names it versions of Microsoft Office 95, 98, 2000, ME, and XP. Make sure that the names match. Also look for version numbers on the box. A version number indicates which software fixes have been included and helps ensure that you get the most up-to-date software with the least number of problems.

Which type of software you purchase usually depends on the type of system used at your facility. Look around, and talk to the people in information services (IS). Find out what they recommend. Do not try to be different. Trying to be different results in problems of compatibility. Incompatible software, such as word processors, creates a situation in which your files may not work with other computers in your facility. Material with which you are dealing electronically (files) may become scrambled or lost in the attempt to move from software to software. The issue of compatibility is also important if you buy software for your home use. Many educators tend to take work home, and if your software at home is not the same, you may be headed for trouble.

One last note: If you purchase software for use in education, it may be possible to get special discounts. However, it is important to note that many of the educational discounts are allowable only if you are part of an educational institution and are not applicable if you work for a health care or other facility. For example, teaching in a school of nursing allows a legitimate discount, but teaching in a staff development department of a hospital may not. This situation varies from institution to institution; check with your IS and legal departments.

5. What is a word processor? How do I learn to use it?

Word processors are the software equivalent of the typewriter. In most institutions, typewriters are no longer available, and the only way you can do your work is by word processor. Few people in the business world continue to use typewriters because of the incredible ability of a word processor to edit and alter content at will. A word processor allows you to type a document, then return to the document and make any changes that may be needed at any point in time. The flexibility of the word processor gives you the power to create class handouts, letters of registration, or class certificates. The word processor gives educators a powerful tool to use as part of the educational process. Of the programs available in the business software packages, the word processor should be the first program that you learn to use. It is also a good idea to start with the word processor because the functions learned for it carry over to the other programs.

Common word processors are Microsoft's Word and Corel's WordPerfect. Many other word processors are available on the market, but these two dominate. Word processor software may be purchased from software vendors, but price ranges vary greatly. Both Word and WordPerfect may be purchased as part of a package in which you receive other programs that can be used for education.

Training for applications such as Word or WordPerfect can be found through a number of resources. If you are interested in taking a class, check with the IS department to see what they recommend. In some institutions, word-processing training is provided by the education department; don't forget to check. If you prefer to go outside of work, check with your local community college or adult education program at the local high school. The training that you want is the same level of training needed by someone looking for an entry-level secretarial job. If you like to study on your own, a wide variety of resources are available, such as video series and books. If you are Internet-literate, consider an on-line course. Dozens of vendors are ready to give you word-processing training at a click. The cost for these courses varies; it pays to shop around.

6. What am I going to do with the word processor now that I know how to use it?

Remember those great handouts that you got at the last conference you attended? How about the newsletter with the staff education schedule? You can create these types of documents in word processor applications. Since many staff educators work with minimal budgets and staff, knowing how to do the typing helps reduce reliance on the department secretary. As you become more comfortable with word-processing, you may find it is easier to type your lecture notes and student notes directly into the computer than to write them first by hand. Converting to this method can be a great time saver. Keep in mind that lectures evolve as they are repeated. With your entire lecture in an electronic format, you can make changes by cutting and pasting instead of retyping. In addition, an electronic document allows you to create student handouts and post-tests directly from the original document.

7. Are there any computer applications that I can use directly in the classroom?

There are several ways in which you can use computer applications in the classroom setting. Graphic presentation programs allow you to produce elaborate presentations of your material and present them directly through the computer. The most popular graphic programs are Microsoft's

PowerPoint and Corel Presentation. These programs, which are included in the business software packages (MS Office and Corel Suite), allow you to create electronic slides, which can be designed with graphics, text, and even video and sound clips.

If you use a graphic presentation program, there are several rules that you want to remember. Any text that you use in your presentation should be between 24 and 36 points, depending on the font type. At this size, participants will find the text easily readable. Keep in mind your audience and the environment in which you are presenting. If you are giving a lecture in a large classroom with a single screen, you may want to make your font a size larger. Along with font size, the type face is very important. These programs may have dozens of font types available, some of which look great but have poor readability. Stick to the standards: Times New Roman, Arial, or Courier New. In terms of slides, color can make a presentation or hamper it. The color of your text versus the background has a profound effect on readability. Using light text on dark background or dark text on a light background improves the readability of the text significantly. Using too many colors in your background distracts participants from the real purpose of the presentation. If you must use multiple colors for text, three colors should be the maximum.

Many special tools can be used within these programs. Some of them can be a tremendous help to your presentation, others a hindrance. Animation capabilities allow your text to appear from nearly any place on the screen. This tool can be highly effective, because it focuses participants on the concept that you are describing while preventing them from moving ahead to the next item. An alternative approach is to put everything on the slide and use a pointer to direct attention to the item that you are discussing. This second technique tends to decrease the number of mouse clicks required during a presentation. Sound effects are also available but tend to be one of the most overused functions. Having your presentation ping, ding, or crash with every change of the screen distracts participants and may lead to loss of connection. Use such functions only when your want to emphasize a point clearly.

Graphics (pictures, characters, objects) are a great way to enhance your presentation, but use them with care. It is easy to find graphics that will work in your presentation. Graphics are included in all of the graphic presentation programs. You can also "grab" graphics from the Internet, but several points should be kept in mind. Many graphics, especially high-quality pictures, are copyrighted and may require a fee for use. Some graphics do not properly translate to specific programs; you may end up with a blurry image. Always give credit to the origin of the graphic in your program, especially if you use medical graphics. Include a footnote at the bottom of the slide with the source information. To find the graphics on the Internet, look for a search engine such as AltaVista, which allows you to search for images only. Let the search engine do the hard work. For health care or medical images, medical image library programs are a great resource. These programs can be purchased from a number of medical publishers. The cost of the programs is significant, but they contain high-quality images.

8. What dangers are involved in using a graphic presentation program?

It is easy to make a great presentation mediocre. Good graphics can help make your presentation come alive, but too many pictures can take away from the content material. In addition, including every word of your presentation material as part of the text tends to bore your audience. They begin to think that you are just reading your notes from the screen. You want your slides to enhance what you are saying and emphasize points as needed.

When you create a presentation, think about what you would enjoy seeing up on a screen. Show your presentation to others before taking it to the classroom. This strategy is especially helpful if you can find people of differing learning styles. Run through the graphic presentation with your verbal presentation at your PC. This technique gives you a chance to make sure that everything fits before you stand in front of a group.

9. Is special equipment needed to use a graphic presentation program?

Yes. This option is not as simple as using overheads. To use a graphic presentation program, you need several pieces of equipment: PC, projector, power source, and screen.

For a PC, it is often preferable to use a laptop. Portability is essential if you plan to take your presentation to different locations. Desktop models can be used if your presentations are frequently held in the same classroom. Also consider using a desktop if you are dealing with budgetary issues. The price difference between a desktop and laptop may be considerable. It is not necessary to look for the most powerful and expensive laptop. If presentations are the primary function of the computer, a machine with a considerably lower cost will suffice.

Besides an adequate processor, the basic requirements for the computer are a 3.5-inch floppy drive, CD-ROM, and video display. The 3.5-inch floppy drive provides you with a way to get your presentation into the computer. Often you may create your presentation on one computer, then transfer it to the laptop. The CD-ROM drive has become a necessity. As you become comfortable with the computer and presentation programs, the size of your presentations will grow. As a result, it takes up more disk space. Using 3.5-inch discs for all presentations is possible, but you may find yourself using multiple disks to load your presentation. Having a CD-ROM allows you to put large presentations on one disk. Writable CDs (using special CD drives that can load your presentation to a CD) are readily available and no longer expensive. If you use guest speakers in the classroom, you may find that having the CD-ROM is the only way to meet their presentation needs.

The last piece of hardware for the PC is the video card. Its importance has more to do with the other piece of equipment that is needed for presentations—the projector. These two pieces of hardware need to be addressed together because their compatibility determines whether or not the presentation works. The projector required is usually called a computer projector or an LCD projector. LCD, which stands for liquid crystal display, is the original technology that provided projection for computer screens. Even though it is an older term, LCD is still frequently used in referring to computer projectors.

The types of currently available projectors are so numerous that it is best to look for information immediately before you are ready to purchase. Looking for information 6 months or 1 year in advance will not provide you with current technical information. What is standard today will no longer be the standard in 6 months. Make sure that whichever projector you purchase or use is compatible with the video card of your computer. The key is resolution (clarity of image), which is defined as the maximal number of displayable pixels in the horizontal and vertical directions. The higher the numbers in each direction (i.e., the more pixels), the sharper the image will be. Ask a technical expert to check the levels of resolution of your laptop's video display, then look for a projector compatible with the highest level of resolution on your screen. Keep in mind that the higher the resolution, the higher the price of the projector. In addition to projectors, many institutions are beginning to use other types of displays, including plasma displays, high-definition television, and flat panel displays.

10. How difficult is it to set up all of this equipment for a presentation?

It really is not difficult at all. Considering that you have spent the past several years caring for patients with complex illnesses and using all of the technology that accompanies such care, you can learn how to set up the necessary equipment. Before you do a presentation, have an expert take you through the steps of setting up. If possible get a set of written directions. Typically there is only one cable, which needs to be hooked up to the video output. Because the cable has a male and a female end, it is impossible to put the ends in the wrong place. In addition, the shape is special so that the cable fits in only one way. A good rule to follow is that you should never need to force a cable plug into place. If you do, you probably ruined your computer. To help alleviate your fears, consider labeling all of the connections. Use matching colors on the connector and the receptacles for the cable. If you use a mouse, you may need to hook it up separately. In some institutions, you may be able to use a network drive to access your presentation. If this is the case, you also need a network card and a network cable.

11. What other programs should the staff educator learn?

As part of your job as a staff educator, you need to manage the education budget and maintain education records. As part of the budgetary process, many institutions use a spreadsheet program. Many spreadsheet programs are available, but the most popular are Excel and Lotus 1-2-3. These programs can help you manage such issues as how much programs cost, including supplies and income that may be received. Using a spreadsheet as a management tool can help you get a quick handle on the costs and benefits of the programs that you produce. Education records are usually kept in a system called a database (see Chapter 16).

A desktop publisher also may come in handy. Microsoft Publisher is the most popular of these programs and can be bought as part of a package deal if you purchase the latest version of Microsoft Office. If you need to decide between saving a few dollars with the cheaper version of MS Office or buying the version with Publisher, go for the Publisher. The benefits are considerable. With a desktop publisher you have access to preformatted newsletters, brochures, letters, and labels. With a publisher you can design sophisticated fliers for your programs, do mailings to both internal and external participants, and create newsletters for the education department. If you happen to have an intranet at your facility, MS Publisher offers the ability to design and create web pages. Desktop publishers are a great way to spice up your work in an education department.

12. How does the Internet help the staff educator?

The Internet can provide help to the staff educator on many levels. The most important is as a resource for information. The Internet can provide you with material on any subject that you may be asked to present. Every staff educator should know how to access and use the various standard Internet resources for health care.

The Internet connects you to databases, which are great research resources. Internet databases may contain information that ranges from full-length articles on a health care topic to a short description of a topic presented at a conference. In either case, it is a lead to more information. To access databases, it is important to learn to use search engines. A wide variety of search engines are available on the Internet. If you already use the Internet, you probably use search engines such as Yahoo!, AltaVista, or Google. In addition, many search engines are specific for health care. They work directly with specific medical or health care–related databases and make valuable resources.

An important database and search engine for nursing, medical, or health care information, is the PubMed system through the National Library of Medicine (NLM). PubMed, which can be found at http://www.ncbi.nlm.nih.gov/PubMed, provides article references that can be taken to a medical library to find hard copy. At some institutions articles may be available through Loansome Doc, an on-line ordering system of the NLM. The other major advantage of PubMed is that it is free. The first time that you use PubMed, take advantage of the tutorial listed on the first page of the website to learn how to use the system to its full potential. PubMed allows you to do most of your content research directly from the Internet.

In addition to PubMed, many other databases of medical and nursing information are available. Some are free, whereas others require a yearly fee. The Medscape (www.medscape.com) database is an excellent resource for medical information. It keeps you informed of the latest developments in health care. Included on the Medscape site is a nursing specialty page. Medscape frequently carries full-length articles. If you are looking for disease-specific information, take a look at the Merck Manual on-line, which can be found at http://www.merck.com. This is the same Merck Manual found in hardback editions, but the on-line version is searchable through a special search engine.

In addition to these medically directed search engines, a few nursing-specific search engines are now available. The American Association of Critical Care Nurses (www.aacn.org), Nursing Center (http://www.nursingcenter.com/), the American Nurses Association (http://www.nursingworld.org/), and Sigma Theta Tau (www.nursingsociety.org) provide search engines leading to nursing-related information. The list of search engines for medicine, nursing, and health care continues to grow. It is important to be on constant lookout for new resources on the Internet.

Other important Internet resources for staff educators, are the web sites of the nursing organizations. Many, if not all of the major nursing organizations now have web sites describing their practice and providing users with access to information about the specialty. An excellent place to start looking is the American Nurses Association site (http://www.nursingworld.org), where you can find links to all of the recognized nursing organizations. In addition to the national organizations, the Internet provides access to local chapters. Many local chapters have now set up their own websites, which can help put you in contact with others in your specialty.

All new staff educators should be aware of the National Nursing Staff Development Organization (NNSDO). The NNSDO website at http://www.nnsdo.org can provide valuable information about upcoming conferences, local chapters, and other resources for the staff educator.

13. How can e-mail be used as a resource for staff educators?

E-mail can be a resource in several ways, depending on what you have at your disposal. If you have access to Internet e-mail either at home or at work, it can be used to access others in the field. If you are new to the field, it is unlikely that you already have contacts. The best place to begin is with discussion lists, or listservs. A listserv or discussion forum is a program that automatically redistributes e-mail to names on a mailing list. You can subscribe to one of these e-mail listservs (or lists for short) by sending a specially formatted e-mail to the list address. Your e-mail address will then be added to the mailing list. You can get information about how to subscribe by looking up the listserv through an Internet search. You can communicate with others who share your interest. Asking for advice or posing a question to a list is a great way to gather information or make contacts for future reference.

The list group that is most specific to staff education is the StaffEdNet list, an electronic mailing list that allows health care education professionals to share and discuss educational issues. Also popular among nursing educators is the NURSINGED list. This group focuses on education from the viewpoint of college educators, but it can be a good resource to staff educators too. Other lists include the JCAHO Watch, Training and Development List, and various lists for clinical specialties. All of these can provide you with experienced contacts who can help with your problems.

14. Can e-mail help with staff education inside the hospital/facility?

Several issues should be assessed if you are considering using e-mail as part of your education process. What kind of e-mail is available? E-mail can range from older character-based systems (with the letters and numbers in green on black) to up-to-date Windows-based systems. The type of e-mail has a major effect on what you can or cannot do. Character-based systems allow only text; you cannot send anything with graphics. However, you can work with a programmer to create specific types of e-mail forms, such as a form for class registrations. If your system is Windows-based, you have a very versatile system. You can send crafted documents with graphics. For example, you can create a document with an update on cardiac disease that contains pictures, diagrams, and whatever else you would like the staff to know about. This document can be sent to hundreds of staff members with a single click, thus eliminating the problems of distributing paper documents. Another way to use e-mail is to send class reminders to registered staff members; this strategy can effectively reduce absenteeism.

There are two possible pitfalls in using e-mail as an educational resource. Do all employees have e-mail, and do they use e-mail regularly? If you do not have e-mail for every employee with whom you work, sending some information by e-mail and some by paper may make the process more complex than necessary. The issue of regular use is a growing concern. Having e-mail does not mean that all staff members will use it. Messages or reminders in e-mail cannot be effective if the staff do not read them. This is a major issue because many staff members are so overwhelmed in their work environment that reading e-mail is their last concern.

Computer Glossary for Educators

Application service provider (ASP): a company that offers access over the Internet to software applications that otherwise would have to be located on the user's own computer. The ASP provides the technical management and housing of the server/database as part of the contract.

Authoring tool: a software application used to create computer-based (CBT) and web-based training (WBT) courses.

Bit: a binary digit.

Browser: a software application used to locate and display web pages. Two common examples are Netscape Navigator and Microsoft Internet Explorer.

Byte: a string of bits (usually eight in modern computers) that represents one character. Amounts of memory are measured in bytes (kilobytes, megabytes, or gigabytes).

CD-ROM: a type of compact disk used to store large amounts of data or programs. A single CD-ROM can store up to 1 gigabyte (GB) of data. CD-ROM stands for compact disk with read-only memory.

Computer-based training (CBT): self-paced education software that allows students to learn by viewing the training program on a computer.

Database (or relational database): an organized collection of related files stored together with minimal duplication. The data in these files can be retrieved through the use of a database application.

DB2: IBM version of a relational database.

Floppy disk: a soft magnetic disk used to transport data or programs from one computer to another. The standard floppy disk today is a 3.5-inch plastic-encased disk. The capacity of a 3.5-inch disk is 1.4 megabytes (MB).

Floppy drive: the drive into which a floppy disk can be placed and run.

Gigabyte: one billion bytes; abbreviated G or GB.

Graphics (pictures, characters, objects): term that collectively describes pictures used in computer programs. It also can be used to describe computer devices or programs that are capable of creating, displaying, or manipulating pictures.

Hard disk: a magnetic disk on which you store computer data. The disk is made of a metal platter coated with magnetic oxide that can be magnetized to represent data. The hard disk is presently measured in megabytes or gigabytes.

Hard drive: the part of the computer that reads and writes data onto a hard disk.

HTML (hyper text markup language): the authoring language used to create documents on the World Wide Web.

Internet: the global network of interconnected computers.

Internet-based training: self-paced training delivered through a browser from an Internet website.

Liquid crystal display (LCD) projector: a device that projects an image directly from a computer. The term is derived from the earliest models, which used a crystal display device placed on an overhead projector.

Learning content management system (LCMS): a system in which computer-based (CBT) and web-based training (WBT) developers can create, store, reuse, manage, and deliver learning content from a central object repository, usually a database. LCMS allows developers to find quickly the text or media needed to build training content.

Learning management system (LMS): software that automates the administration of training events. All LMSs manage the log-in of registered users, manage course catalogs, record data from learners, and provide reports to management.

Listserv or discussion forum: allows people to communicate about various topics by posting messages and replies to messages under the heading of a particular topic. A collection of messages and replies about a topic is often referred to as a *thread*. Listservs are not chat applications in which people exchange typed messages in real time.

Megabyte: one million (1,048,576 to be exact) bytes, the unit most commonly used to describe the amount of memory or data storage capacity. Megabyte is abbreviated M or MB.

Monitor: the display screen. The term usually refers to the hardware that includes the housing for the screen's electronic components and the stand on which it tilts and swivels.

Network: two or more computer systems linked together.

Network card or network interface card: a circuit board that is inserted into a PC to allow it to send and receive information from a network.

Oracle: the world's leading supplier of relational databases. Oracle databases are used in most large database systems.

Pixel: a single dot in the picture on a computer display screen.

Processor or central processing unit (CPU): the silicon chip that executes stored program instructions. There are typically two components to the CPU, the arithmetic logic unit (ALU) and the control unit. The ALU performs arithmetic and logical operations, whereas the control unit extracts instructions from memory, then decodes and executes them.

Random access memory (RAM): a type of computer memory that can be accessed randomly. Any byte of memory can be accessed without touching the preceding bytes. RAM is commonly found in computers, printers, and other devices. It is also used to describe the main memory of a device and the amount of memory available to programs. Most PCs have at least 32 megabytes of RAM.

Resolution: the clarity of the computer display screen.

Search engine: a program that searches documents on the World Wide Web for specified keywords.

Spreadsheet: a table of values arranged in rows and columns; also used to refer to the applications that allow you to create and manipulate spreadsheets on the computer.

SQL Server: a relational database developed and marketed by Microsoft corporation.

Writable CD, CD-R, or CD-RW: a special type of compact disc on which data can be erased and overwritten by new data; a popular back-up method.

Web-based training (WBT): any type of education in which the student learns by connecting to a program on the Internet or intranet. These programs are written in one of the web languages, such as HTML.

Word processor: a program or computer that enables you to perform word-processing functions, such as creating, editing, formatting, storing, retrieving, and printing text.

Video card or video adaptor: the board that plugs into a PC to give it display capabilities. The quality of the display depends on both the adaptor and the monitor itself.

World Wide Web (WWW): a system of Internet servers that support documents in HTML. Not all Internet servers are part of the WWW.

BIBLIOGRAPHY

1. Capron H: Computers: Tools for an Information Age, 6th ed. New York, Addison-Wesley, 1999.
2. Gookin D: Word 2000 for Windows for Dummies. New York, Hungry Minds, 1999.
3. Hall B (on-line): available at www.brandon-hall.com.
4. Harvey G: Excel 2000 for Windows for Dummies. New York, Hungry Minds, 1999.
5. Levine J, et al: Internet for Dummies, 8th ed. New York, Hungry Minds, 2002.
6. Lowe D, Jasmine G: PowerPoint 2000 for Windows for Dummies. New York, Hungry Minds, 1999.
7. Saba V, McCormick K: Essentials of Computers for Nurses: Informatics for the New Millennium, 3rd ed. New York, McGraw-Hill, 2001.
8. www.webopedia.com Darien, CT, INT Media Group.

6. STAFF DEVELOPMENT DEPARTMENT MANAGEMENT

Diann C. Cooper, MSN, RNC, *and Jean M. Bulmer*, MSN, RNC

1. Discuss various ways in which a staff development department may be structured.

A nursing staff development department may be organized in a variety of ways. One way is to consider the types of customers to be served. Staff may provide services to (1) nursing exclusively; (2) to a larger scope, such as all patient care areas; (3) to all staff within a given organization; or (4) to all staff of a corporation that is located at several sites and provides several levels of care. The table below illustrates how a department may be organized based on the types of customers served. Reporting structures in nursing staff development departments may be visualized in a similar way.

	CUSTOMERS	POSSIBLE REPORTING RELATIONSHIPS	FOCUS
Level 1	Nursing staff	Nursing administrator	Clinical skill development
Level 2	Clinical staff	Administrator or service leader	↓
Level 3	All staff in organization	Vice president (VP)	
Level 4	All staff in a corporation	Executive VP or VP for education	Competencies, organizational development

Clinical focus also depends on how the department is structured. A department that serves nursing staff may have a primary focus on clinical skill development, whereas a department that provides services to multisite or multicare levels may focus on ensuring competencies and organizational development.

2. What is the benefit of assigning liaison responsibilities to education staff members?

Choosing or assigning a liaison is an important decision. Liaisons function as the contact point for the education department. Often these relationships are established because of the staff development person's interests, specialty, or experience. The benefits can be many. If the liaison has been included in the planning sessions for the department, the needs of that department are known beyond its own membership. If the department identifies an additional need at a later date, members know whom to contact. When liaison assignments are based on specialty or interest, the department has a certain level of comfort, knowing that the liaison can relate to its needs or concerns. The liaison relationship helps promote the feeling that members of the department are special: they have a liaison and a priority focus. Liaison relationships also provide the foundation for networking relationships. They allow liaisons and department members to strike up a conversation at general meetings, "hallway meetings," and even national organization meetings or seminars. Needs that are identified by surveys or other forms can be communicated to departments by the liaison. Needs that are identified by other education department members can be communicated to the appropriate department's liaison, who can follow up with members of the department.

3. What process should be used for handling program requests?

Requests that come into the education department can be delegated to the requesting department's liaison. It is important to follow these requests informally because they may represent a more generalized, house-wide need. If a house-wide need is identified, the department as a whole must decide who will take on the request. You may wish to consider the following factors:

- Who has the time
- Who is the "expert" in the requested area
- Who has an interest in the material
- Who has the experience

These requests may require the attention of more than one person. Some departments may choose to assign requests. Other departments may choose to discuss them at their staff meeting or via e-mail or other messaging system. Your department secretary, if you have one, is often the first person to receive such requests. He or she may be able to direct some calls to the appropriate liaison without going through the meeting process.

4. Why are department missions, visions, and goals important? How do I develop them?

All departments should have a mission, vision, and goals. These statements provide a purpose and direction for all activities and serve as a guide for how you operate your department. All projects or activities should be considered in terms of how they will achieve the department's mission, vision, and goals. If the activity does not contribute to their achievement, there is little reason to pursue it.

A department's mission, vision, and goals should support and contribute to the organization's mission, vision, goals. The first step is to consider your organization's mission, vision, and goals. With that information in mind, create department-focused statements. Review your mission and vision annually; review and revise goals quarterly. For example:

Organization's vision:	To excel in patient care delivery
Organization's mission:	To meet the health care needs of our patients
Strategic goal:	To ensure optimal patient outcomes
Department vision:	To excel in education and staff development
Department mission:	To meet the educational needs of staff who serve our patients
Strategic goals:	To assess and ensure staff competency
	To provide regular training in new technologies
	To monitor errors and incidents and to provide training to improve patient outcomes

5. How can I show that staff development is making a difference? That the department is making a difference?

Pretests and posttests can demonstrate an increase in knowledge. Reduction in errors can be measured after a training program is completed. Cost savings may be measured after a training program that highlights the costs and correct use of certain patient care products.

Staff development department effectiveness may be measured by gathering data about staff satisfaction with the department's services, by calculating the number of employees who were trained in a 1-year period, the number of hours of training per employee per year, or the training costs per employee (see Chapter 17).

6. Describe ways of measuring productivity.

One way is to ask each staff member to record information about the services that they have provided during the month. For example, they might record the program title, date, duration, and number of participants (see sample data collection sheet in Appendix A).

In addition to classroom training, other activities can be recorded, such as the development of learning materials (posters, self-study booklets), time spent in coaching a staff member, and consulting services. These values can be tracked on a monthly basis and observed for trends as well as included in an annual report to administration (see example on following page).

The Saratoga Institute (www.SaratogaInstitute.com) publishes an annual report that can be used to benchmark training productivity with those of different industries as well as with health care organizations of various sizes. Data are reported in a number of ways, including the number of hours of training per employee and the training cost per employee. *Training* magazine also periodically publishes productivity data in its monthly magazine.

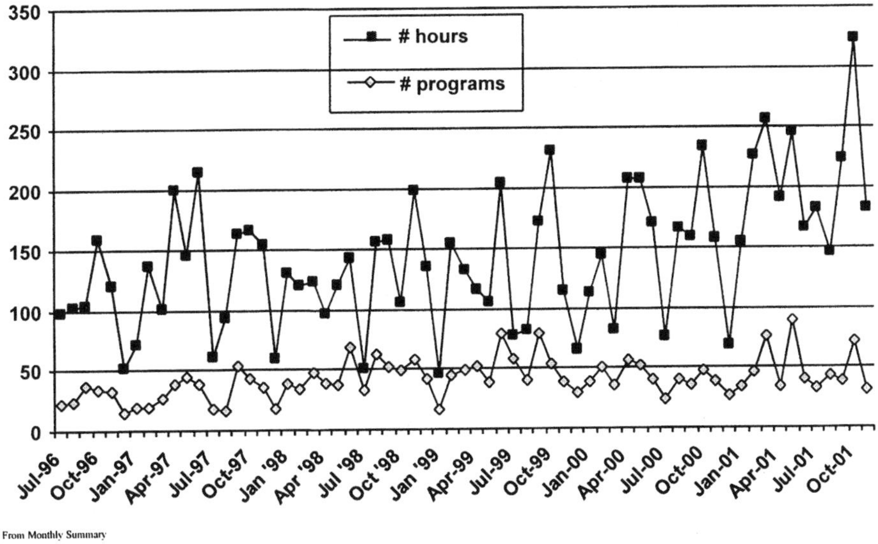

Education department activity.

7. What data can I use to stay focused and efficient without going crazy?

Look at your list of things to do. The items that support your organization's goals and objectives, affect the organization as a whole, or affect patient care should become your priorities. Try to determine which ones can be accomplished quickly and which ones will require more planning. Ponder your list: Are any items on the list *not* educational needs? Are there any items that cannot be "fixed" with education? Make certain that the identified needs are truly needs and not wants. Focus on items that make employees more effective in their job. Consider needs that are supported by quality assurance monitoring data, risk management (incident report) data, and other institutional reports. Look for ways to provide education to meet the need in the most appropriate manner. Needs that are unique to a certain department may be best met by a teleconference or a self-learning packet rather than a huge, day-long seminar.

8. What should be included in a staff development budget?

The items in a budget can vary greatly, depending on the size and scope of your department. The following items may need to be included in your budget:

- Salary
- Refreshments/food and supplies related to these items
- Training/demonstration supplies (e.g., IV bags and tubing, tape and dressings)
- Office supplies (e.g., paper, pens, pencils, markers, flip chart paper, folders)
- Photography and slides, photocopying, binding, specialty printing/paper costs and services
- Books, booklets, videos, software, magazine subscriptions
- Teleconference fees
- Speaker honoraria and travel costs
- Tuition and scholarship funds
- Memberships/dues
- Travel and registration fees (for department member's education)
- Minor equipment (e.g., to replace old or broken flip charts, overheads, slide trays)
- Maintenance agreements
- Lease agreements (e.g., for computers, fax machines, copiers)
- Telephone, postage
- Equipment maintenance costs

9. How is managing a staff development department different from managing a direct patient care department?

Management of a staff development department is significantly different from management of a patient care department. Primary customers are usually employees as opposed to patients. A key function is to provide support and services to the customer—to the staff. The staff development department needs to maintain close connections with its customers to be aware of educational needs and to act quickly to meet those needs. It also needs to maintain connections with other areas throughout the organization (e.g., quality assurance, safety, administration, accreditation, medical education). These connections provide a dual purpose. First, they help keep the department connected to issues, problems, and changes across the organization. The staff development department can then anticipate and respond to changes with training programs for its customers. Second, these connections enable the department to provide input into policies and decisions throughout the organization.

10. Our department recently moved away from the main hospital. As a nurse and an educator, I am having difficulty with being off-site. What can I do?

As systems grow, off-site locations become more and more common. As with any change, you need to find ways to do the work of your department differently to meet the needs of your customers. Areas to explore include how to get materials to class participants before courses begin, how to maintain visibility and still get work done, how to arrange meetings and schedule to allow adequate travel time as well as adequate and timely communication, and how to stay connected.

Question 10 in Chapter 3 deals with bridging the gap between education and nursing. A move to an off-site location is another variable that may contribute to this gap. Brainstorm within your department for ways to improve your visibility and connectedness to the people you serve. You must make a concerted effort to place yourself with your customers (the staff) and to meet their needs. Your role in education is to support the staff. An off-site location makes this goal hard to accomplish, but it is possible to make the best of it.

Hint: Decorate your office in a way that you like and provide a positive, happy, safe environment. It is your home away from home and your refuge when the going gets tough.

11. How should staff development records be maintained? What documents should be kept and for how long?

Staff development records can be maintained in an electronic format or a paper file. The e-format may take more time to enter data, but the advantages are that it takes much less space and data retrieval can be much faster. Files may be arranged chronologically, alphabetically, or by topic area. Chronologic arrangement facilitates filing and removing old records. Alphabetic or topical arrangement may make records easy to find if there is consistency in how you name and categorize your records. If consistency is lacking (such as naming a file "Basic Arrhythmia Course" vs. "ECG course"), finding records may be more difficult.

The contents of staff development records can vary and may include information such as program advertising (flyers), sign-in sheet/attendance lists (see sample in Appendix B), handouts, presenter information, equipment lists, room set-up information, expense/revenue information, pre- and posttest scores, and an evaluation summary.

Records should be kept for 3–5 years, depending on the type of program. Programs that have contact hour credit must be kept for 5 years; other program records may be discarded after 3 years. Certainly you can keep records longer than the time frames suggested above. Space is sometimes limited, and in departments that offer a high volume of programs, there may be no place to store records indefinitely. Remember to back-up (make copies of) your electronic files frequently.

12. What policies may be needed for a staff development department?

You may wish to establish some policies for commonly asked questions or items that require a standard answer. Examples include fees for programs, tuition for classes, registration process, cancellation of classes, use of classrooms, quality assurance and monitoring, confidentiality, resolving disputes, and instructor responsibilities. The policies that you need may depend on the size and responsibilities of the department (see sample policy in Appendix C).

13. What strategic or annual program planning should be done by the staff development department? How can it be done?

At least once a year, a staff development department should get together to do strategic planning. The group should evaluate its mission, vision, and goals to ensure that they are still in alignment with the organization's mission, vision, and goals. This assessment should be followed by a review of services and discussion about how to improve or redesign service delivery. Your group should ask the following questions:

- What should be added, deleted, or done differently in light of changes to the organizational or departmental mission, vision, and goals?
- What changes are needed in response to new accreditation requirements or changes in organization size or services?
- What are the department's strengths, weaknesses, opportunities, and threats?
- What actions should be taken in response to this assessment?
- What tools are needed for the department to function better and more efficiently?
- What roadblocks interfere with doing our job?
- What do our customers say? (review survey results, program feedback information)

After a department analysis is completed, program plans for the upcoming year may be made, perhaps selecting dates for orientation, cardiopulmonary resuscitation, advanced cardiac life support, or other regularly scheduled courses. Announcements of these program dates can be made to department managers so that employees can be scheduled and other events can be planned so that they do not conflict.

14. What should be covered at a monthly staff meeting?

Monthly staff meetings are an important way to stay in touch with the other members of the department. Staff meetings should be organized, with an agenda, start time, and end time (see the sample meeting agenda form in Appendix D). To develop a sense of camaraderie, you may wish to bring in bagels for breakfast or to celebrate a birthday at the beginning of the meeting. The agenda should include items such as the following:

- Budget (requests or reports of status)
- Program updates (who needs help, who is teaching what)
- Program planning and goal setting
- Choosing liaisons
- Yearly planning of programs
- Staff time off/vacation requests

15. How can I boost the image of the education department?

Image is important. The education department is often in a position of influence, but not always power. It is in that challenging gray area between staff and management. As a result, it is important to develop an image. To develop or boost your image, consider the following ideas:

- Chose a name with strength and influence. Perhaps your organization has "centers of excellence" or "strategic business units." Consider how you can take advantage of these names for the education department.
- Discuss how you want your course flyers to look. Some information should remain the same regardless of who develops it. Your name, phone number for registration, the ADA statement, and the statement about food should be consistent.
- Your materials should be of high quality. Make certain that you use spell checks and grammar checks on the items that you create.
- Use an auto response on your e-mail that includes your title (staff development specialist) and the name of your department.

- Dress appropriately. Keep your clothes neat and in line with your organization. You never have a second chance to make a first impression.
- Be professional in your conduct. Keep your cool when you are confronted with a conflict. Stay away from questionable jokes or language.
- Keep your department professional in appearance. Create the atmosphere of a "corporate university." Chose your office arrangements with comfort and professionalism in mind. Have chairs available for customers who are waiting. Use plants and pictures to create an atmosphere. If you have dedicated training space, use some posters to inspire and some for reference. Take a customer service course to learn how to respond to customers in person and on the phone.
- Create a registration book and registration phone line. Answer voicemail quickly (even if it is just to say, "I'll get back to you on Monday").
- Be reliable. Under-promise and over-deliver—but always deliver.

16. What ideas may be helpful for streamlining registration, evaluation, flyers, and other processes?

Registration is important because it allows you to plan the amount of supplies and materials that you will need. However, registration by telephone takes a lot of time. A registration voice-mail line allows people to register without tying up your telephone line.

Flyers can be streamlined by creating one flyer and saving it. The date and time can be changed the next time the course is offered. If you have more than one person in the department, you may wish to create a "share drive." Computers can be networked and a common drive created so that flyers, policies, and work plans do not need to be re-created. Evaluation forms can be tallied on a share drive by creating an Access database. Generic evaluation forms can be used for programs that are not regular offerings. Specific evaluations can be created, saved, and modified later. A file drawer in a cabinet can be set aside for the most current copy of a self-learning packet, policy, program handout, or other material. Then, instead of recreating the material, you can pull it out of the file and have it copied.

Appendix A: Productivity Report, Hamot Medical Center, Center for Education and Staff Development (used with permission)

Month:__________________

Title	Date	Time	Total # times offered	Length of one session (in hours)	# attendees	# RNs	# Contact hrs	Instructor	Reason Code	Comments, or **reason for canceling**

Use this page to record the completion of "Enduring Materials." Enduring Materials are products that have a potentially wide audience and can be used repeatedly. Record the information only once, at the time when the product is ready for use. Examples: creation of a harassment self-learning packet, revision of the back safety poster, development of a customer service survey on 4 South, "Nursing at Hamot" Game, a self-test to measure stress levels.

Description of the Material Created	Purpose when or how it will be used	Target Audience	Creator (from CESD)	Reason

Reason codes
1. inservice (Hamot specific)
2. continuing education (applicable beyond HHF)
3. orientation
4. mandatory
5. addresses performance improvement
6. advances in science and technology
7. evaluations from a class
8. committee recommendation
9. manager request
10. consultant recommendation
11. previously identified need
12. commnity involvement/outreach activity (professional)
13. community involvement/outreach activity (nonprofessional)

Appendix B: Attendance Record

Title: ______________________________ Speaker: ____________________
Program date: ____________ Time ____________ Place: ____________________
Fee: __________ Contact hour ______ CESD contact: ______________ Code ______

NAME	POSITION/TITLE	DEPARTMENT
1.		
2.		
3.		
4.		
5.		
6.		
7.		
8.		
9.		
10.		
11.		
12.		
13.		
14.		
15.		
16.		
17.		
18.		
19.		
20.		
21.		
22.		
23.		
24.		
25.		

From Hamot Medical Center, Erie, PA (used with permission).

Appendix C: Sample Policy

DATES: Effective January 2001
Reviewed January 2001
Revised

TITLE: Course Cancellation Policy

I. PURPOSE: To establish guidelines for canceling programs sponsored by education services.

II. POLICY STATEMENT: Education Services is committed to providing quality, cost-effective education to all WellSpan participants. All efforts will be made to ensure timely, effective notification of all participants when course cancellations occur due to inclement weather, low enrollment, or other unanticipated events.

III. EQUIPMENT:
E-mail course cancellation notice
Phone course cancellation notice

Participant course cancellation letters
Education Services Course Cancellation Notice

IV. PROCEDURE

A. Course Cancellation Decisions and Notifications

1. Course cancellation decisions are made on a course by course basis.
2. Courses generally require 6 to 8 participants for cost-effective adequate group exercises and interactions. Courses with low enrollment may be cancelled the week prior to the course date. All participants should be notified a week prior to the scheduled date and every effort made to work with participants to find alternative solutions.
   Exceptions to this policy include New Nursing Employee Orientation (NNEO), Nursing Assistant and Unit Secretary courses. In these courses, Education Services will work with Human Resources to tailor the program and work with Human Resources to meet participant needs.
3. Participants should be notified at least a week in advance of the cancellation whenever possible. Personal contact should be a priority to ensure the person has received the cancellation notice. Participants can be notified by phone and e-mail and through managers as an additional resource. When personal contact is not possible, ask participants for a response back in all cases to ensure they receive the cancellation notice in a timely manner. Cancellation contact processes should be coordinated and confirmed by the Education Specialist and Administrative Assistant responsible for the program.
4. Immediately upon cancellation, the room reservation should be erased from the schedule book and media services called to cancel any AV equipment and service previously scheduled for the course.
   A course cancellation notice should be completed and placed at the front desk. This includes the course title, date, time, room number, facilitator or contact person's name and number, reason for cancellation, alternative options such as future course dates and times, a list of participants and how they were notified of the cancellation and when they were notified.

B. Inclement Weather Cancellations

1. Anticipated cancellations due to snow or ice will be discussed the day prior to the program and a plan initiated to address all programs with a 9 am or earlier start time.
2. Cancellation decisions are made by the facilitator of the program with involvement from Team Leaders or the Director of Education Services. In cases where a judgement call is needed, decisions should err on the side of safety for participants and instructors as well as consider staffing needs in patient care areas. Facilitators should work with team leaders to help verify this.
3. Decisions for all programs with afternoon start times will be deferred until the next morning. A plan will be devised to address possible cancellations due to weather conditions.
4. Facilitators, Team Leaders and the Director of Education Services will coordinate a plan to address cancellations from home if necessary and should be prepared with course rosters, participant names and numbers and a WellSpan Directory. Follow processes outlined in the Course Cancellation Decisions and Notification section of this policy.
5. Unanticipated weather changes may require a revised plan.
6. The Director of Education Services will notify department Team Leaders of any declared snow emergencies.

V. DOCUMENTATION

Document cancellation notice in e-mail / letters.
Written cancellation notice at the front desk at reception area.

VI. APPLIES TO: PERSONS PERMITTED TO PERFORM:

Education Services Director (responsible for cancellation decision)
Education Team Leader (responsible for cancellation decision)
Education Specialist (responsible for cancellation decision)
Administrative Assistants

VII. AREA PERFORMED:

Education Services

VIII. REFERENCES / RESOURCES:

N/A

From Wellspan Health, York PA (used with permission).

Appendix D: Staff Development Meeting Agenda/Record, Hamot Medical Center, Erie, PA (used with permission).

1. Meeting Date: ____________ 2. Time ____________ 3. Location ____________

4. Attendees: [ ] ________ [ ] ________ [ ] ________ [ ] ________ [ ] ________

Others attending:

Topic:	Main Points:	Decision/Conclusions:	Next Steps:
Topic:	Main Points:	Decision/Conclusions:	Next Steps:
Topic:	Main Points:	Decision/Conclusions:	Next Steps:

5. Future File (items for further discussion, but not for this meeting)

6. Next meeting: Date: ________ Time: ________ Location: ____________

Agenda:

-
-
-
-

____

Signature of Recorder

7. LEGAL AND ETHICAL ISSUES IN EDUCATION

Kristen L. O'*Shea*, MS, RN, *and Cheryl* B. *Robinson*, MSN, RN

1. What ethical issues arise in education?

Although the issues that may face you as an educator are not the "life-and-death" issues of clinical areas, ethical issues arise whenever choices are made. Ethics deals with the principles governing ideal or good behavior. Ethics focuses on why a behavior is right or wrong. A good example of an ethical issue in education is whether or not to seek funding from a pharmaceutical company for support of an educational offering. On one hand, the company will fund a renowned speaker to come to your facility. On the other hand, the motivation of the pharmaceutical company may be to encourage your hospital to use its particular medications. In a perfect world, you would have all the money that you need to bring in the best speakers without the pharmaceutical company. Unfortunately, such is not the case, and you are faced with a dilemma.

The dilemmas that educators face in their jobs tend to fall within the realm of a branch of ethics known as organizational or administrative ethics. Unfortunately for you, the ethical issues that you learned about in nursing school deal with biomedical ethics. Organizational ethics deals with the conflicts and tensions "created by differences in organizational, individual and professional values."[1] Examples of organizational ethical dilemmas facing educators include how to respond to cheating, confidentiality conflicts, falsification of records to meet standards, and a variety of other thankfully uncommon challenges.

2. What should I do when I am faced by an ethical dilemma?

A decision-making process should be used to evaluate ethical issues carefully. The first step is simple acknowledgement of the ethical issue. In some cases, because of the busy nature of our lives, you simply do not see that an ethical conflict or issue is involved. In the case of organizational ethics, these situations are not life-and-death issues, but they can affect greatly the integrity and character of your department or institution. Simply acknowledging the existence of an ethical conflict, a situation in which a person is faced with a decision that may be incongruent with the organization's values or policy, is an important first step.

Secondly, it is important to clarify the nature of the conflict. Write out a statement of the problem. The next step is to identify the issues or processes that are involved in or responsible for the conflict. Then it is important to identify the possible alternatives or solutions for resolving the issue. As part of a team, you should solicit help from your colleagues in brainstorming the possibilities. Lastly, you should select and implement a course of action.

3. What resources are available to me in dealing with issues such as these?

In dealing with issues that come up, it is important that you include others to help you. Consider using the expertise of your manager or even your vice president in helping you to sort out the issues related to the ethical dilemma you are having. Look to the leadership of your organization to help you with issues such as these. It is important that others who work in your department have a chance to share how they have dealt with similar issues in the past and be involved in solving your problem.

Several documents help provide a framework for evaluation of ethical issues. You can look to the American Nurses Association's Code of Ethics for Nurses. You can be find the major provisions of the Code on-line at www.nursingworld.org/ethics/chcode.htm. Hospitals often have mission, vision, and value statements that provide a framework for important decisions. Similarly, some hospitals have adopted a "code of conduct" that employees sign at the time of hiring. This document helps employees know where the hospital stands regarding "right" behavior. Examples of statements from a code of conduct include:

- Conduct all activities with integrity, honesty, respect, fairness, and good faith in a manner that reflects positively on our health system and its affiliates.
- Maintain the confidentiality of privileged business and personal information.
- Be truthful in all forms of professional and organizational communications, and take steps to avoid or stop the dissemination of information that is false, misleading, and deceptive.

Statements such as these help to guide your decisions in dealing with ethical issues.

4. Should I accept money from pharmaceutical companies to fund educational offerings?

It depends. Pharmaceutical companies offer a great service to medical and clinical education by providing funds for offerings. As a department, you must decide whether you will seek pharmaceutical support for education and what rules you will follow to ensure ethical behavior. Most institutions have statements forbidding the acceptance of gifts or money with the expectation of influencing a decision related to purchase of products. Accrediting bodies, such as American Nursing Credentialing Body and the American Medical Society, require full disclosure of speakers' interests to the audience before speaking engagements. Effort should be made to minimize potential bias. Speakers should ensure objectivity and balance in their discussions. You need to keep all parties involved in the program focused on the promotion of learner knowledge rather than promotion of commercial products.

5. What is one of the most common ethical or legal issues that I will face?

Confidentiality issues are probably the most common type of conflicts. Personnel information, such as grades on a test or performance on a competency evaluation, is considered confidential. An employee's personal information is also considered confidential. You must understand that you may be privy to confidential information and be constantly aware with whom you share it. Release of information has legal as well as ethical ramifications.

Another confidentiality issue in the educational setting is patient information. You must not use patient names or other identifying information when you discuss a case in class, and you must make sure that the patient's name is removed from any materials that you have copied for the purpose of educating staff. There is no doubt that copies of monitor strips tell a real story and provide an excellent teaching opportunity. Just be sure that the patient's right to confidentiality is not breached.

6. A staff nurse recently received a poor grade in one of my courses. How and when should confidentiality be protected?

First, consider who is asking for the information and why he or she needs to know. Does the person have a legitimate right to know? Pretest and posttest scores as well as general attendance information may be considered confidential material. If people attend an educational program on their own time, their successful or unsuccessful participation does not need to be shared with their employer. Permission to release information should be requested. If the employer has paid for the nurse's attendance, it is appropriate to share attendance as well as class performance with the nurse's manager. This information should not be shared with other staff unless they have a responsibility relative to the supervision and evaluation of the nurse.

7. A new nurse told me that she is being treated negatively by staff. She asked me not to say anything to anyone. What should I do?

This is a common problem. Educators are often perceived as "safe." We are easy to confide in, and we are not "management." You are truly walking a fine line in this case. You have a responsibility to influence the retention and morale of the nurse. On the other hand, she has asked for confidentiality. How you handle this issue is important. It can have great impact not only on the new nurse but also on your credibility with other staff. You need to find ways to help on both sides of the equation.

You should talk to the new nurse and brainstorm possible solutions. Ask for permission to discuss the issue with the nurse manager, if she is unwilling to do so herself. Gently persuade her by showing how dealing with problems can make improvements in the work environment. It may be that a particular unit is not the right one for this particular nurse. Your coaching and guidance can make a big difference in the start of the nurse's work life.

8. I was shocked to learn that nurses were simply copying the answer sheet to a self-learning packet test that I wrote and submitting it for credit. What should I do?

It is truly disappointing when professionals cheat. Cheating is a breach of integrity and is contrary to almost every ethical code, whether it is Code of Ethics for Nurses or your hospital's value statements. Does your hospital have a specific policy for testing and cheating? Most do not. In any case, it is difficult to deal with situations such as these.

The first step is to be sure that you have the whole story. Carefully discuss the matter privately and individually with the nurses involved. If indeed cheating occurred, you must decide with your manager what steps will be taken. It may be difficult in the case of self-learning to determine what in fact took place. You need to proceed carefully. Consult your human resources department, and use the problem-solving process described in question 2.

9. How can I prevent cheating?

Cheating while taking an exam in a classroom setting can be partly prevented by removing opportunities. Structures such as ample spacing between participants, limiting personal effects, and proctoring decrease cheating on exams.

Consider placing a statement on your self-learning packets confirming that the module was completed by the person who submits it, such as "All participants completing the self-learning packet agree to complete it independently without collaborating or receiving answers by other means. Participants agree that all work has been completed by the person receiving credit."

Cheating occurs only when you expect the person to take a test. Be sure that you need to evaluate the person with a test. At times testing is appropriate, but it is not the only way to evaluate knowledge.

Ample evidence indicates that high school and college students cheat. Such evidence is disturbing in regard to nursing students because it raises questions of integrity. Staff nurses may have participated in a culture of cheating in college. Staff development departments should have a zero tolerance policy in relation to cheating in conjunction with a statement about academic integrity and operational definitions of cheating. Some people actually believe that it is acceptable to cheat! Be clear about what educational activities and evaluations are individual work and which allow collaboration. Also consider writing a statement about the penalties for cheating.

10. What if I suspect that a class participant is under the influence of alcohol or drugs?

Most health care institutions have strong policies against the unauthorized use and sale of alcohol and drugs in the workplace. Two points are important to assess. First, what are the behaviors of the participant? Second, is the participant attending the class as a requirement of employment? Your health care institution should have specific steps that you must follow if the participant is attending on paid time and his or her behavior is suspicious. You have a responsibility to take reasonable action to prevent participants from harming patients, people in your classroom, or themselves. The list of behaviors that you may notice includes the following:

- Stumbling, staggering, or falling when walking
- Swaying when standing
- Shouting, slow or slurred speech
- Use of profanity or belligerent language
- Crying
- Excessive sleepiness
- Bloodshot, glassy eyes
- Alcohol on breath
- Fumbling movements

If you see a combination of these behaviors, you should remove the employee to a private spot and review your concerns. If, after talking with the employee, you believe that he or she is impaired, you should follow your institution's policy. It may involve an evaluation by employee health or the emergency department. Be sure to document what happened.

11. I have been asked to backdate documentation of a department's completion of mandatory education requirements by a few days so that they can meet regulatory compliance. What should I do?

Clearly, falsification of records is unethical behavior. Using the problem-solving approach described in question 2, determine the issues and processes involved with this problem. If your education department is off-site and relies on mail service, this request may be reasonable. What is reasonable behavior? If staff have simply missed the deadline, you must document the completion as you would on any other day.

Such requests challenge your moral code. With these requests and issues come opportunities for quality improvement as well. Further investigation of issues and problem-solving can lead to improvements that prevent such requests in the future.

12. Am I at risk to be sued if a nurse whom I educated does something wrong?

Nurses are licensed professionals and are responsible for their own actions. Be sure, however, that your training materials are up to date. Information that is provided during orientation and inservices can be considered information that the nurse is responsible for knowing and implementing. For example, it is possible for attorneys to request training materials and attendance records from an inservice to show that a nurse has received information on a given topic.

As an educator, if you are aware that a staff nurse is not competent and do not try to correct the situation, you may be held individually liable if the staff nurse commits an error.

13. What can I use to determine correct practice?

Nurses are responsible for knowing the standards and policies that affect their practice. The American Nurses Association provides "Standards of Clinical Nursing Practice" that set the minimal requirements for acceptable practice. In addition, nurses should be aware of the standards set by national professional nursing organizations as well as state nurse practice acts. Hospital policies and procedures should be based on national standards and reflect the current practice at your hospital. Of interest, failure to follow the hospital's procedure is the one of the most frequent legal finding against nurses.

14. What should I know as an educator about the Americans with Disabilities Act (ADA)?

The ADA provides the right to equal access to programming and training to people with physical, psychological, and learning disabilities. You, as a nurse educator, need to know that some of your students are protected under this law. It is up to you to determine how to provide education (see Chapter 13).

15. What is the copyright law?

US Code: Title 17 is the copyright law. This law protects original work. As an educator, you need to know that you must give credit to the original author of any work that you use in the classroom or in written format.

16. Can I make copies of articles for a class that I teach?

The US Code: Title 17, Chapter 1, Section 107 defines "fair use" of copyrighted materials. Multiple copies for classroom use are not considered an infringement of copyright.

US Code: Title 17, Chapter 1, Section 107: Limitations on exclusive rights: Fair use

Notwithstanding the provisions of sections 106 and 106A, the fair use of a copyrighted work, including such use by reproduction in copies or phonorecords or by any other means specified by that section, for purposes such as criticism, comment, news reporting, teaching (including multiple copies for classroom use), scholarship, or research, is not an infringement of copyright. In determining whether the use made of a work in any particular case is a fair use, the factors to be considered shall include:

(1) the purpose and character of the use, including whether such use is of a commercial nature or is for nonprofit educational purposes;

(2) the nature of the copyrighted work;

(3) the amount and substantiality of the portion used in relation to the copyrighted work as a whole; and

(4) the effect of the use upon the potential market for or value of the copyrighted work.

The fact that a work is unpublished shall not itself bar a finding of fair use if such finding is made upon consideration of all the above factors.

BIBLIOGRAPHY

1. Badzek LA, et al: Administrative Ethics and Confidentiality Privacy Issues. Available at www.nursingworld.org/ojin/topic8/topic8_2.htm, p 2.
2. Rostant DM, Cady RF: Liability Issues in Perinatal Nursing. Philadelphia, J.B. Lippincott, 1999.
3. Silva MC: Organizational and Administrative Ethics in Health Care: An Ethics Gap. Available at www.nursingworld.org/ojin/topic8/topic8_1.htm.

II. Planning Issues

8. NEEDS ASSESSMENT

Diann C. Cooper, MSN, RNC

Identifying learning needs is an important activity for the staff development specialist. Before you plan a program, you should know whether or not the program is needed. The way to find out is to perform a needs assessment.

1. What is a needs assessment?

According to *Webster's Dictionary*, a **need** is "a condition marked by the lack of something requisite." A **needs assessment** is the process of identifying what is missing. The missing pieces may help people perform the job at the required level or even higher. Although the literature contains many different definitions of needs assessment, the author believes that it represents the first step in the educational process. Like the first chapter of a book, it sets the stage; it identifies the main characters and gives an idea of the story line. A needs assessment identifies the learning need and the area to which it is related. This point is important: the needs you wish to address in your educational program are learning needs. Often a needs assessment identifies other needs, such as performance, personal, and human needs. **Performance needs** refer to how the person performs his or her job. A performance need is related to a roadblock in the work setting; the person knows how to perform but cannot or chooses not to do so. A **personal need** is related to the person's interest and desire to learn about something that will not be used on the job. A **human need** is related to Maslow's hierarchy of needs: safety, security, belonging, and self-fulfillment. Personal, performance, and human needs are important, but you should not spend the majority of your time in planning to fulfill them. Some of these types of needs can be met in other ways.

2. What are some of the advantages and disadvantages of a needs assessment?

If you have children, you probably have taken them to a friend's house for a birthday party or some other get-together. Have you ever tried to find the house without good directions? Have you gotten lost as a result? A needs assessment is an important "map" to help you meet the actual learning need. Advantages and disadvantages of needs assessments include the following:

Advantages

- Needs assessments provide data from the learners themselves.
- The data can help you identify needs that cross departments or units.
- The information can act as a "pretest" and characterize the situation before you intervene.
- Needs assessments support promotion of a particular program to a particular department.
- Needs assessments make people aware of discrepancies and their importance.
- By identifying the discrepancy, learners may be more motivated to learn about the topic.
- Needs assessments help staff development departments set priorities as to which classes should be offered first and what resources should be allocated to each class.
- The data provided by needs assessment can be either broad or specific, depending on the design of the assessment.
- Needs assessments allow staff development departments to take a proactive role.

Disadvantages

- Learners may not know or be able to identify what they truly need to know.
- Needs assessments are valid for a short period; they need to be repeated.

- Many staff development personnel have not been taught how to put together a needs assessment or how to analyze the results.
- Needs assessments can be labor- or time-intensive (surveying a sample of 2500 employees requires sending out and receiving 250 surveys).
- Needs assessments are seen as educational research. Research often scares people and is seen as dry, difficult, or boring.
- Learners may assume that if the needs assessment is not creative or interesting, the classes will not be either.

3. Why should I do a needs assessment?

Mailloux said it well: "a learning needs assessment provides the rationale for the expenditure of millions of dollars to plan and present educational programs for nurses."[9] The first step to program planning is identification of a need. Program planning is a key staff development activity. The programs are important to a variety of customers, from certification bodies who need to ensure that nurses remain competent in performing their role to the nurses themselves as they seek quality educational programs. Needs assessments identify needs that are current and thus ensure that your programs are timely.

Needs assessments are often the focus of a staff development department. They provide objective data that support why a program was offered and demonstrate the activity level of the department. By providing programs that are pertinent and timely, your department is seen as reliable, supportive, and responsive to the needs of the staff and organization. This is a major benefit for any department. On a smaller scale, a needs assessment can provide the data that you need to enlist an individual manager's support for a program. Objective data from an accurate needs assessment demonstrate to the manager your commitment to his or her staff.

4. How do I put together a needs assessment?

That is a big question that is best answered by dividing it into smaller, more manageable pieces: underlying assumptions, choice of focus, the three levels of assessment, the six steps in conducting an assessment, and methods of gathering information.

5. What assumptions guide a needs assessment?

Four assumptions have been identified in the literature[13]:

1. The first assumption is that the staff can identify their learning needs. According to this assumption, performance, personal, or humans needs are identified. Occasionally the learners do not see a need that has been identified by direct observation, quality assurance/improvement reports or other activities (some of which are discussed later).

2. The second assumption is that conditions are always changing. As mentioned above, needs assessments are not valid for a long period. Change occurs quickly; what was a need this week may not be next week. As a result, needs assessments must be an ongoing process. It is important to use a variety of methods so that your needs assessment remains as up to date as possible.

3. A third assumption is that by identifying learning needs, you can identify outcomes. If the identified needs fall within the psychomotor domain, for example, the outcome will include demonstration of a skill by the educator followed by demonstration of the same skill by the learners. A cognitive domain deficit can be demonstrated by a pretest. After the course is completed, a posttest can be administered to demonstrate that learning occurred. A need in the affective domain can be much harder to measure.

4. The fourth assumption is the importance of involving more than one person in the process of identifying needs. As Williams[13] states, "multiple view points will aid in accurately identifying the leaning needs of a particular group." The choice is yours.

6. How do I choose a focus for my assessment?

You may want to begin by asking this question: Are you trying to identify orientation, inservice, or continuing education needs? Orientation is an important part of the activities of any staff development department. Although orientation is an expectation for every new employee, each new employee has a different need for orientation. The length of time spent on a topic will vary from person to person, depending on individual need. Inservice needs relate to the requirements for a particular job. As new policies, procedures, and equipment are implemented, the need for an inservice program arises. Inservice needs are constantly changing as job responsibilities change. Continuing education needs are associated with employees' interest in expanding their knowledge base or career interests. They are more than what is needed to perform the job at the expected level.

7. What are the three levels of needs assessment?

Needs assessments have been classified as focusing on three levels: organization, job or task, and individual employee or person. It has been suggested that needs assessment should start at the organizational level to determine whether a need exists and what organizational factors contribute to its existence. Then the jobs, work, or tasks should be examined to identify performance issues (i.e., what tasks are not being performed). Lastly, the individual employees are assessed to determine what learning needs must be met for the tasks to be performed and organizational needs fulfilled.[6]

The author finds it helpful to ask the following questions: Is this assessment designed to identify the needs of a particular group (such as a certain department)? Or is it designed to be a business-wide assessment? Am I trying to find a common theme throughout the organization or just among the most experienced nurses? It is important to consider what you think you are looking for.

8. What are the six steps in conducting a needs assessment?

Step 1: Answer the "why" question. Why do I believe that a needs assessment is necessary? What do I hope to discover? What effect will the future program have on this group?

Step 2: Decide who has an interest in the assessment. Does the manager need to be involved? How about human resources or quality assessment? Or does the interested group consist of experienced preceptors? Ponder this question carefully. Sometimes the author pulls together a small group to begin the process and asks who else needs to be included. You also may call people on the phone, discuss the idea briefly, and ask them who should be included in the first meeting. You do not want to leave out key players. If you do, the success of the program may be prevented.

Step 3: Determine who can help with the needs assessment. Do you have a secretary who will type it? If not, who can? To what location will the surveys be returned? Who can help tally them? Consider the costs and time involved. Will you need to pay someone to help you?

Step 4: Chose a method that works best for the focus of your needs assessment. Some methods are listed later in the chapter. You want to chose the most cost-effective method that suits your focus. During this step, you create the questions that you will ask if you conduct a survey or a focus group or the items that you need from quality assurance or other data reports.

Step 5: Conduct the needs assessment.

Step 6: Analyze the results, and share them with your original planning group. At that meeting you should begin to establish your priorities (see below).

9. How do I get the information I want or need?

Now that you have established the "who" and the "what," pick the "how." Some methods can be divided into categories such as primary, secondary, or combined sources and high use, moderate use, or low use. Needs assessment techniques also can be viewed as research and divided into various research categories. The format that you choose depends on the group for which you are attempting to identify needs. Possible methods include the following:

- Survey
- Benchmarking
- Interviews
- Focus group
- Committees
- Observation
- Records and reports
- Job descriptions
- Performance appraisals
- Personnel records
- Checklists
- Advisory groups
- Professional standards
- Tests
- Changes
- Process recording
- Organization mission/vision statements
- Industry data
- Review of the literature
- Delphi technique
- Nominal group process
- Slip technique

10. When should I use a survey?

Surveys (questionnaires or opinionaires) are common. They consist of a series of questions that ask readers their opinion on a topic. Surveys are great tools to use when you want to obtain information from a large group of people. For example, patient satisfaction surveys are sent to all patients, and customer surveys are sent to all customers. You can use a survey to ask all staff members in a particular unit about their learning needs. It is an easy way to ask the same questions of all the people and get anonymous responses. Surveys also can be conducted over the telephone, although the effectiveness of this approach may be changing. (See Appendix A for an example of a needs assessment survey).

11. How do I develop a survey?

Surveys are divided into sections. The first section contains questions that describe the person responding to the survey (e.g., age, sex, years worked in a unit or profession, educational level). These questions help you to understand the "typical" respondent.

The body of the survey contains questions related to the content about which you hope to gain more knowledge. It may include questions about orientation, inservices (policies, equipment), or continuing education (further development of skills). Your planning group can help you determine what questions to ask. Survey questions may be written in open-ended, close-ended, or sentence-completion (fill-in-the-blank) formats. The number of questions varies. One minute per question is the accepted standard.

You need to establish a rating scale for the survey. Consider how you want the reader to respond. Is a "yes" or "no" response adequate, or do you need a Likert-type scale? A Likert scale is the most common choice, with 1 and 5 representing opposite ends of the spectrum (i.e. ,1 is the least and 5 is the most of something). Although the 1–5 Likert scale is common, it is not uncommon to use an even number of possible responses. This strategy prevents people from choosing the neutral answer (usually 3 on a 5 point scale). The respondents who tend to chose a neutral answer are required to chose one that is slightly to the "most" or slightly to the "least" end of the scale. This approach provides more information about the topic. It can add strength to your survey and the identified needs if the majority of the answers are on the "least" end of the scale. You may wish to use words that represent opposite ends of a dichotomy, such as "good" vs. "bad" or "fair" vs. "unfair." These scales also can be represented by a line with a word at each end. The respondents are instructed to place a mark on the line indicating their position.

12. What is benchmarking?

A benchmark, according to *Webster's Dictionary*, is "a marked point of known or assumed elevation from which other elevations may be established." Benchmarks in health care are often comparisons between organizations or data, with one being the accepted expert. Some organizations pay a fee to be included in a database that allows them to compare themselves with other organizations of similar size. Such comparisons are often anonymous; no actual identifying data are available in the database. The only identifying characteristics are bed size, acute vs. chronic care, patient acuity, specialty, or the like. These figures can be quite helpful in trying to decide whether the response for your hospital is "good enough."

13. Is interviewing staff helpful?

Interviews are a great way to get in-depth points of view. They allow the opportunity to dig more deeply, to explore questions and clarify items. You can conduct an interview with anyone. The type of information that you are seeking determines whom you should interview. For example, if you are exploring the needs of nurses on a particular unit, you want to select a novice nurse, a competent nurse, an expert nurse, and representative nurses from the different shifts. If the hospital has a clinical ladder, you can interview one nurse from each level. The nurse manager of the unit can assist you in selecting people to interview. Person-to-person interviewing allows relationship-building between colleagues. Such relationships can be essential when you reach the program planning stage.

14. How do I set up an interview?

Interviews can be structured or unstructured. Unstructured interviews begin with a general question and flow from there, based on the responses. A structured interview consists of a specified list of questions to be covered. Questions can be closed- or open-ended, or a combination can be used.

15. What is a focus group?

A focus group is a powerful information-gathering technique that uses small group discussion to identify the views of people in the group about a certain subject. Focus groups are helpful in gathering perceptions about a defined area of interest. The group discussion provides data and insight that other data collection techniques do not. Focus groups bring together a group of people for 60–90 minutes. A leader and an observer have prepared relevant questions ahead of time. The leader asks the questions, and the observer documents verbal and nonverbal reactions of participants. Sometimes focus group discussions are recorded so that the observer can focus on the nonverbal reactions and tone of the discussion. The answers provide a better understanding of the interests of your customers. Groups are usually small (5–9 people). Development of a nonthreatening, comfortable atmosphere is important. Some discussion is allowed during the focus group.

16. Can hospital committees be a source of information?

Yes. Often a committee can identify needs. Staff members may approach committees with requests for programs, which can be shared with you. They also may have observed behaviors related to a learning need or performance deficit. Committees such as patient safety, quality assurance, and medical records review have access to interesting information that may identify significant learning needs. The advisory group is a related method of needs assessment.

17. The nursing units are quite busy. How can I find out their learning needs?

Observation can be an effective method to use on busy nursing units and gives the educator an opportunity to validate information provided by others.[4] This approach, however, takes some planning before you sit and observe. When you decide to gather data by observing others, you need to establish ahead of time exactly what you are going to observe. For example, perhaps you are curious as to why so many cardiovascular patients have postoperative infections. You decide to visit the cardiac surgery units to observe when and how many times the staff wash their hands. Observation can provide you with objective data about how policies and procedures are implemented, how well patient care is documented, whether equipment is used or not, and much more.

18. How can I incorporate quality assurance and incident reports into a needs assessment?

Such reports are a major source of information. Quality assurance tracks many issues and has lots of data. Incident reports tell us when and where mistakes occurred. Look for trends. Ask yourself, "When did this incident occur? On a certain shift? On a certain day of the week? In a certain unit? With a particular piece of equipment or patient population? With a certain medication?" These questions help determine whether a trend is present and whether it is related to something else. Quality assurance data are based on actual practice and reported on a monthly basis. These reports are tabulated, and trends over time can be easily identified. Often the reports gather data about items that were contained in previous incident reports or identified by other methods. Quality assurance data represent the follow-up that occurs when deviations from standards of practice or care have been identified and corrections implemented.

19. Who else in the hospital can help determine needs?

You may wish to talk with many people about needs. Infection control may help identify a disease transmission trend. The safety committee can provide data about the number of slips and trips, back or neck injuries, fires, or thefts and department responses. Perhaps one department did not respond appropriately to a fire drill on an off shift. A review of the policy and procedure may be needed. Course evaluation forms may list potential topics that reflect learning needs. Their widespread use and familiarity also may make the data more acceptable to other members of the organization.

20. What other documents should I consider in identification of needs?

The following documents are available at your health care organization but may be less helpful in identification of needs:

Job descriptions list the expected abilities of people in a particular role. Combined with observation or another method, they may help identify a discrepancy between ideal and actual practice.

Performance appraisals often are within the realm of the human resources department, which may have a database with a great deal of information about the number of people who need assistance and why or the number of higher performers. You may be able to obtain the top five or so reasons for poor, average, or above-average performance. The average age of performers (or years of service, department, shift) also may be included in this database. If you work in a hospital accredited by the Joint Commission for the Accreditation of Healthcare Organizations (JCAHO), this organization also prepares a report to the board of directors. The report contains some of the same information listed above and can be a good source of needs identification, or it can be used to report how well the identified needs from the previous year were met. This approach is also called "position analysis."

Personnel records can be helpful if you are trying to identify the needs of a particular group. Managers often have files filled with little notes about a number of issues. To be the most beneficial, the material should be objective with clear, succinct descriptions of situations or behaviors. These "tickler files" or "anecdotal notes" can be reviewed for trends. You can pick a specific period of time and look for common themes in the files. These themes then can be supported with data from other sources, such as those listed previously. Most managers will not let their tickler files out of sight, so you may have to review them under the manager's watchful eye (and probably in his or her office).

Checklists may have been used in orientation programs and with competencies to help ensure that all of the content is covered. You can review these checklists for trends. For example, you may review the orientation checklists of all new graduates hired within the past 6 months to determine whether they all request or identify the same learning need. If they do, you can proactively add this need to the orientation program for future graduates. Checklists can be used during brainstorming sessions to help the group identify needs. You can ask members of the group to list their top five learning needs. You also can use them to narrow the need if it is too general. For example, perhaps a group identified "computers" as a need. You can use a checklist to determine whether the need involves an inpatient computer system, the Internet, or use of databases or office programs. The information identified on a checklist can be ranked from lowest to highest to help you set priorities.

21. What are advisory groups?

An advisory group is a group of people who represent the target audience for a program. The people may be from within the organization, from outside the organization, or a combination of the two. The group should be small (around 8 people) and should meet at regular intervals. Advisory groups can be helpful in identifying topics and speakers for programs. They focus on identified needs and discuss creative ways to meet those needs. In large organizations, several advisory boards may be in place, each with a different focus (e.g., oncology, critical care, trauma, patient education).

22. Many groups have established professional standards. How can they help me?

Professional standards represent the expected performance of people in a certain group. These standards may be associated with professional groups, specialties, or accreditation groups. They are not used so much to identify learning needs as to serve as the benchmark against which individual performance is evaluated. When a discrepancy exists, a learning need has been identified. It is a good idea to be familiar with the professional standards of your specialty group.

23. Are tests helpful in identifying learning needs?

Pretests and posttests can help to identify a need and to ensure that the program fulfilled that need. In other words, pretests determine what you already know about a subject, and posttests determine what you learned as a result of the course (or what the teacher taught you). This is a simplified approach to a much more complex topic—question development. Tests take time to develop and should be assessed for validity and reliability. As a result, the tests used before and after a course may provide information about items that the instructor was not able to teach effectively and should be examined carefully to determine whether they truly reflect the learner's acquisition of knowledge.

24. Health care changes so quickly. Can these changes be a source of learning needs?

Definitely. Changes in services, equipment, and procedures represent learning needs. As computers become more a part of everyday life, the changes that they represent can indicate a potential learning need. With the advent of the Internet and, for some institutions, the intranet, many staff may have had limited (or no) experience with this technology. Any change represents a potential learning need.

25. Can other industries help to identify health care needs?

It is a good idea to watch industries other than health care. Industry data are related to benchmarking and reviewing the literature. New educational trends and activities may arrive in other industries before they reach the hospital. Often you can be proactive and begin your data collection with this thought in mind. For example, the postal industry and schools have instituted programs to prevent violence. Health care is just starting to take action against violence. You can be proactive by assessing where you stand now.

26. What is a review of the literature?

A review of the literature helps to identify current issues and future possibilities. Look at what is going on around you. Review more than just one journal per month. Look at journals from other specialties, including non-nursing or non–health care journals. You may find interesting data in editorials, websites, on-line journals, and articles in newspapers. These data can be used to support other identified needs, or they can be stepping stones into bigger needs assessment projects.

27. What research methods can help me determine needs?

The Delphi technique and Nominal Group Process are used to obtain consensus and priority. The **Delphi technique** involves mailing questionnaires to a specific group of people. When the questionnaires are returned, the responses are summarized and the questionnaire refined. A revised questionnaire is sent to the same group of people for further input. This process allows the select group of people to arrive at consensus by frequently ranking and reranking their responses. This process can be time-consuming; if time is an issue, it may not be the ideal method to choose.

Nominal Group Process requires bringing together a select group instead of mailing surveys. Once the group is present in a room, the facilitator asks the members to identify their needs within a certain subject or topic area. Each person states one need. No discussion of the identified needs takes place, unless a brief definition or description is needed to clarify a statement. When everyone has had a chance to speak and no other needs can be identified, the listed needs are ranked in order of priority (from highest to lowest or most important to least important). Each person is expected to rank the items on the list. Eventually this process results in a list of needs that is created through consensus and ranked in order of priority. Although the process takes about 2 hours and can be very helpful, it can also limit creativity and brainstorming because it is highly structured and does not allow discussion.

28. Explain the slip technique.

The slip technique is similar to the Nominal Group Process. The difference is that the information is written on a slip of paper that each person submits. This technique can be likened to the secret ballot. Each person has a stack of paper or 3×5 cards. After a question or problem is posed, each person writes down one answer on the slip of paper and turns it in to the facilitator of the group. The slips of paper are then read and tallied. The same process of ranking and determining priority that is used with the Nominal Group technique can be implemented. Facilitators are reminded to hold onto the slips of paper. Do not throw them away in front of the participants, because it shows lack of respect for their opinions.

29. Are certain methods more appropriate for one situation than another?

Yes. Process recordings are most helpful in identifying learning needs related to communication. Process recordings "may consist of verbatim report of a conversation recorded by another or they may be recorded by the nurse after the conversation."[15] Such recordings can memorialize an event with objective information and can be helpful in dealing with an angry patient or family. Review of these recordings can identify needs related to interpersonal communication.

30. Who can help me perform needs assessment?

As mentioned above, you should involve people who have a vested interest in the identification of needs. You also should look to the planning department, quality assessment department, or perhaps the person responsible for research. These resources can help you organize your thoughts and questions as you develop the needs assessment tool. They also may have additional information to support needs identification.

It is also wise to include a member of the management team for the department with whom you are working to identify needs. You will need this person's support once the needs are identified and the program is planned. You may want representatives from the group of people whose needs you are assessing. If you are trying to identify the skills used by nurses on the cardiac unit, you may want to include a few of those nurses in the creation and review of the tool that you plan to use. You also should keep your supervisor informed about your activities with this group. He or she may be able to tell you of other activities with the same group or with a related group that may affect your plans. Perhaps, for example, members of the cardiac unit are being surveyed already for their opinion about a new telemetry monitoring system. You may need to adjust the telemetry-related items in your needs assessment. If you are new to the process of needs assessment, you may want to ask a colleague in another department who has used needs assessments in general or the method you have chosen in particular to review your plan before you begin. This person may be able to provide information about pitfalls to avoid or other suggestions that will aid in the success of your needs assessment.

31. Once I have the data, how do I know that a specific need is real?

When the same need shows up in a variety of sources, it is likely to be real. When patient-controlled analgesia (PCA) pumps are identified on a survey and an evaluation form and the quality assurance report identifies the number-one medication error for the past month as PCA pumps, the need for PCA education is more valid than if it appeared on only one of these items. Consider the response rate. If you used a survey or questionnaire as your needs assessment method, how many of them were returned? How many were properly filled out? Although it is difficult to identify an actual number needed for significance, one author states that the "greater the number of responses, the more reflective the findings are."[15] Also consider how broad or narrow your focus was. Were you looking at the needs of the organization or the individual?

32. What is the difference between an interest and a need?

You definitely want to focus your energies on the educational need, although you should not ignore completely the identified interest. Educational interests reflect a learner's desires or preferences for learning. These interests may not be related to the learner's job or responsibilities. Perceived educational needs are the learner's perceptions about the need for instruction in a particular area. Again, they may not be related to the learner's role in the organization. Learners may not always be aware of all of their learning needs. True educational needs can be met through some form of education. They may or may not be perceived as educational needs. True educational needs have the following characteristics:

1. They are identified by multiple methods.
2. They are found in needs assessments with a good response rate.
3. They follow the focus (if your focus was individual, your assessment has identified individual needs).
4. The needs can be addressed by educational methods.
5. The needs can improve performance (they are related to the individual's role within the organization).

33. I have identified hundreds of needs. How do I set priorities?

Setting priorities involves looking at the identified needs and considering which should be addressed. In many staff development departments, financial and staff resources are often spread thin. Priorities must be appropriate to the situation, realistic in relation to the demands of nursing and patient care, and feasible both financially and in terms of time.[1] Needs that receive your first attention may involve "life-and-death" issues (code blue training, PCA pumps). Some needs represent key hospital services (e.g., admissions, same-day surgery). Others have priority because they are related to practice changes or new equipment. Others may be pressing needs for a particular unit or department. To establish priorities, involve the same people who helped plan the needs assessment. Also involve your fellow department members. Often, your customers know which needs should be addressed first.

34. What do I do with the information that I have gathered? With whom do I share it?

Your needs assessment should be reported and shared with the same people included in the planning stage. If you included members of the planning department, they may have already developed a format for reporting the data revealed by your needs assessment. They will enter the data into a computer program that provides you with a report broken down into different categories. The report may include additional variables (e.g., years of experience in the unit).

35. What should I document in a needs assessment report?

If your planning department does not have a preestablished format or if you do not have a planning department, you may wish to consult the literature. Consider inclusion of the following:

- Summary by position (numbers of active staff, questionnaires distributed, percentage returned)
- Summary by position and division (e.g., RNs, PCA)
- Summary by position of demographic data
- Listing by position of "other" data and comments from the demographic sheet (importance and motivation ratings)
- Mean and medians for importance of each topic and motivational ratings for each topic
- Summary by position and division of categories and topics with the top three ratings (include importance and motivation)
- Names of people interested in presenting programs or suggested speakers and topics

When the report is ready, you will want to share it with the group who helped you plan the assessment and the group with the vested interest. You also may want to share it with your supervisor. When you share the information, be prepared to help the group make important decisions. Priorities need to be set as to which educational needs are to be addressed and in what order. Below are suggested questions:

- What problem needs to be solved?
- Will education correct the problem?
- Who needs the education?
- What are the consequences of not providing the training or education?
- What are the comparative benefits of the different offerings that may be presented?
- What are the motivational levels for the needs?
- What training is available from other sources?[11]

This is the beginning of program planning, which is covered in the next chapter.

36. How long is the information valid?

Needs assessments are not valid for long periods. The needs that you identify are current needs. As change occurs, the needs may no longer be valid. It has been reported that current technology will be outdated in 5 years. The more specific your needs assessment, the shorter the time it is valid. For specific needs assessments, it is best to try to meet a short list of top needs (for example, the top 3–5). Your needs assessment may have to be repeated in 6 months to 1 year, depending on focus and specificity. A needs assessment done by your staff development department may provide enough information to allow planning for 1 year. Such planning is considered timely and on target. If you use an annual needs assessment survey, you may want to consider conducting a focus group or a series of interviews at the 6-month mark to determine whether there has been a drastic change. You can use your planning group, another group, or an advisory committee to help with this task. A discussion with the supervisor of the area with which you are working is also crucial. He or she may have an idea of what changes are building on the horizon or if things have been stable. The process that we discussed earlier begins again (also called ongoing needs assessment).

37. How can I do a quick needs assessment?

For people who are in single-person departments or who work primarily as clinicians at the bedside, formal needs assessments can be next to impossible. However, determining that a need exists is still important. You can do a quick needs assessment at staff or committee meetings. If you have e-mail, send a message to a group of people and ask them to answer one question. Use your unit's quality assurance data or other reports that come your manager's way. If you are a bedside clinician, you will use observation as your most common method of needs assessment. You know by watching whether staff have a difficult time with a procedure or particular type of patient. Confirm that observation by discussing it at a staff meeting or looking at infection control reports. Be creative. The information is available; it simply has not been examined.

38. Do I need to do a formal needs assessment?

No. Formal needs assessments refer to the more time- and labor-intensive methods, such as surveys, focus groups, and research techniques (e.g., Delphi techniques). Use what has already been created or gathered. Do not attempt to reinvent the wheel! Use available committees, quality assurance reports, incident reports, patient safety reports, and other data that are already handy. Always look at more than one source, however. The more often the same need is identified, the more valid it is.

39. What is the difference between systemwide and unit-specific needs assessment?

Systemwide needs assessments can be a good idea if one has not been done for a while (if ever). You need to seek information from a large number of people who represent the overall staff of your organization. To do so means looking at your organization to determine percentages (e.g., the number of people in each department, in certain age groups, with a certain number of years of experience, with management experience). You want the group with whom you work to represent as closely as possible the entire group. This is not an easy task. Usually, a systemwide assessment is not done alone. It can be quite helpful in determining overall needs and needs that cross departments.

Unit- or department-specific assessments are designed with a particular department in mind. They focus on the customers served and the equipment or skills needed to work in that area. The results may not be applicable to other areas. Unit-specific assessments, however, may point to potential problems elsewhere. For example, if one department cannot properly check a certain piece of equipment, perhaps other departments have the same problem. The author uses department-specific assessments more often than systemwide assessments.

40. What are some of the common mistakes in doing a needs assessment?

You will not live long enough to make all of the mistakes yourself; learn from the mistakes of others. Below are some tips to keep in mind as you try your hand at needs assessments:

- Choose your focus carefully. Try not to duplicate the work that someone else has just done. It skews your results and makes people question your motives.
- If you use information from another source, give the source credit.
- The fact that it shows up on your survey does not make it a need. Look carefully at how you originally wrote the question. Perhaps you led people to the response that they gave.
- Remember the KISS rule: Keep It Short and Simple. Long and difficult surveys lose the audience quickly. Your assessment is no good if no one participates.
- Managers do not always believe you. Just as learners do not always identify their learning needs, managers do not always agree with the needs identified by their staff. They want to look competent, and if your assessment identifies a need by which they feel threatened, they may not accept it. Look for another answer. Be creative. Find support in another department. Verify the need with another method. Instead of a large-scale program, develop a monthly newsletter for staff and address the need in the newsletter

Learning needs assessment is an important staff development activity. Needs assessments are like a road map to a friend's house; without them you do not know which direction to go. Start off simply; you may want to look at the last program you put together and ask yourself, "How did I know this program was needed?" You may find that assessing needs is easier than you thought.

BIBLIOGRAPHY

1. Alspach JG: Needs assessment. In The Educational Process in Nursing Staff Development. St. Louis, Mosby, 1995.
2. Apgar C: Making it count: Key factors to consider when assessing continuing professional educational offers. J Trauma Nurs 1:6–14, 1999.
3. Chatham MA: Discrepancies in learning needs assessments: Whose needs are being assessed? J Contin Educ Nurs 5:18–22, 1979.
4. Courtemanche BM: Determining educational needs of staff nurses: An assessment tool for nurse educators. J Contin Educ Nurs 3:104–108, 1995.
5. Gillette N: Focus groups: How to make them work for you! Program Participant Manual. Pittsburgh, PA, VHA Pennsylvania, 2000, p 2.
6. Holton EF: A snapshot of needs assessment. In Phillips JJ, Holton EF (eds): Conducting Needs Assessment. Alexandria, VA, American Society for Training and Development, 1995, pp 1–12.
7. Jazwiec RM: Learning needs assessment. Part I: Concepts and process. J Nurs Staff Devel 2:91–94, 1991.
8. Jazwiec RM: Learning needs assessment. Part II: Methods. J Nurs Staff Devel 3:138–142, 1991.
9. Mailloux JP: Learning needs assessments: Definitions, techniques, and self-perceived abilities of the hospital-based nurse educator. J Contin Educ Nurs 1:40–45, 1998.
10. Morrison RS, Peoples L: Using focus group methodology in nursing. J Contin Educ Nurs 2:62–95, 1999.
11. Panno JM: A systematic approach for assessing learning needs. J Nurs Staff Devel 6:269–273, 1992.
12. Punch KF, Horner B: Stages in the development of a needs assessment questionnaire. J Nurs Staff Devel 4:176–180, 1991.
13. Williams ML: Making the most of leaning needs assessments. J Nurs Staff Devel 3:137–142, 1998.
14. Yoder-Wise PS: Learning needs assessment. In Abruzzese RS (ed): Nursing Staff Development: Strategies for Success. St. Louis, Mosby, 1992, pp 183–202.

Appendix A: Education Survey

1. At which facility do you work?
   - ☐ Hamot Medical Center
   - ☐ Immediate Care
   - ☐ Imaging Center
   - ☐ Forestview/Springhill
   - ☐ Physician Office
   - ☐ CPFG
   - ☐ Other, please specify: ______________________________
2. In which department or unit do you work? ______________________
3. What shift do you usually work?
   ☐ Days ☐ Evenings ☐ Nights ☐ Rotating shifts
4. Are you: ☐ Full-time ☐ Part-time (I or II) ☐ Per diem
5. What days of the week do you *usually* work?
   ☐ Monday–Friday ☐ Saturday-Sunday ☐ Rotating
6. How difficult is it for you to attend programs during work hours?
   ☐ Very difficult ☐ Somewhat difficult ☐ Not difficult
7. How difficult is it for you to attend programs on your own time?
   ☐ Very difficult ☐ Somewhat difficult ☐ Not difficult
8. How likely would you be to attend an education program?
   a. In the morning _____ very likely ____ somewhat likely ____ unlikely
   b. During lunch _____ very likely ____ somewhat likely ____ unlikely
   c. In the afternoon _____ very likely ____ somewhat likely ____ unlikely
   d. During dinner _____ very likely ____ somewhat likely ____ unlikely
   e. At night _____ very likely ____ somewhat likely ____ unlikely
   f. In the evening _____ very likely ____ somewhat likely ____ unlikely
   g. During a break _____ very likely ____ somewhat likely ____ unlikely
   h. No time is good _____ very likely ____ somewhat likely ____ unlikely
   i. Other, please specify ______________________________
9. How likely would you be to attend an education program that was:
   a. 30 minutes _____ very likely ____ somewhat likely ____ unlikely
   b. 45 minutes _____ very likely ____ somewhat likely ____ unlikely
   c. 1 hour _____ very likely ____ somewhat likely ____ unlikely
   d. 2 hours _____ very likely ____ somewhat likely ____ unlikely
   e. 4 hours _____ very likely ____ somewhat likely ____ unlikely
   f. 8 hours _____ very likely ____ somewhat likely ____ unlikely
   g. Other, please specify ______________________________
10. How likely would you be to attend an education program that was:
    a. In a conference room at Hamot (main campus)
    ______ very likely ____ somewhat likely ____ unlikely
    b. In my department/worksite
    _____ very likely ____ somewhat likely ____ unlikely
    c. Off site (at a hotel or conference center)
    _____ very likely ____ somewhat likely ____ unlikely
    d. Other, please specify: ______________________________
11. How do you prefer to learn new information?
    - ☐ Attend a class
    - ☐ Watch a videotape
    - ☐ Read a journal article
    - ☐ Complete a self-learning packet
    - ☐ Computer-assisted learning
    - ☐ Other, please specify: ______________
12. How do you find out about the education programs offered at Hamot?
    ☐ It's Friday ☐ Flyers ☐ Co-workers ☐ E-mail
    ☐ Bulletin Boards ☐ Manager ☐ Education Calendar
13. Please list some *job-related skill development programs* you would like the education department to sponsor (for example, treatment of heart attacks or accessing e-mail):
    ____
    ____
    ____

14. Please list some *health care issues* that you would like to hear about (for example, managed care, confidentiality of information, case management, or gene therapy):
____
____
____
15. Are there any *personal development* topics that would be of interest to you (for example, dealing with change, communication skills, or delegation skills)?
____
____
____
16. How does your manager assist you to meet your educational needs? (choose all that apply)
   - ☐ Grants me time off to attend programs
   - ☐ Pays for some (or all) of program expenses
   - ☐ Notifies me of educational opportunities
   - ☐ Other: ______________________
17. What suggestions do you have to make education more accessible to you?
____
____
____

From Hamot Hospital, Erie, PA (used with permission).

9. PROGRAM PLANNING

Jean M. *Bulmer*, MSN, RNC

1. What is the first step in program planning?

There are actually two steps to take before moving full speed ahead with planning a program. First, determine the need for the program (see Chapter 8). If there is not a bona fide need for the program, you may be wasting your time and effort. Second, you need to know your target audience.

- *Find out their background and level of experience.* A program geared to a novice will be quite different from a program for experienced practitioners. A program for physicians can be quite different from a program for nurses.
- *Determine preferred learning styles.* Does your target audience prefer lectures, computer learning, hands-on experiences, or independent study? Consider their age and realize that younger generations may have a greater comfort level with computer instruction, whereas older adults may be more used to lectures.
- *Assess motivation to learn.* Find out if continuing education is required for their license or certification or if are they seeking new skills so that they can advance in their field.
- *Determine how easy is it for them to attend an education program.* Can they get away during work time—or do they prefer to attend programs after work hours or on a day off? Find out if there are better times of the day or days of the week for them to attend a program.

Failure to know your audience and their needs may result in lack of interest in your program.

2. Who should be involved in planning an education program?

Program planning may require one or two people or a large group. The number of people involved depends on the program topic, length, and complexity. Full-day seminars may require a number of people; a unit-based education program may be organized by a unit educator alone.

3. What do I need to do to plan an education program for my unit?

Once you have determined the need for a program and your target audience, your next steps are to select a speaker; determine the date, time, and location of the program; and then advertise the program. Allow yourself 1–2 weeks. Appendix A contains a checklist for various activities.

4. How do I select the speaker?

Choose a speaker who is an expert in the subject matter. Other important considerations may be travel and fees for your speaker (if any), ability to present the topic according to the teaching method that you have identified, teaching skill of the speaker, and ability of the speaker to present the information at a level appropriate for your target audience. You may want to get references from others about the skill of the speaker, view a tape, or observe a presentation before you make your decision. Once you select the speaker, it is important that you tell him or her how the need was assessed, your target audience, objectives, and preferred teaching methods. Specific information for the speaker may be put in a confirmation letter and/or a speaker contract and/or a speaker information form (Appendices B, C, D, and E). Confirmation letters and contracts should be done for a full-day conference but may be optional for a small unit-based program.

5. How do I determine the best date and time?

Sometimes the date of a program depends on the availability of the speaker. National speakers often schedule their engagements 6 months to 1 year in advance. This is important to know when planning a full-day conference. Local or internal speakers may need only 1–2 weeks' notice.

You also need to consider your audience when choosing the date. Some clinical areas may be busier and staffing may be higher on certain days of the week than others. Mondays and

Fridays are sometimes avoided because of their proximity to the weekend. Staff may "forget" about a Monday program (if they were off for the weekend) or may not want to go to a Friday program because their mind is focused on weekend activities. Certain times of the day also may be better or worse, depending again on the unit. Avoid times when there will be numerous admissions, discharges, procedures, or medications to be administered. Don't forget to consider what other events may be going on (e.g., other education programs, internal celebrations, holidays). Your best course of action is to ask the target audience which day and time are best for them.

6. How do I decide on the location?

When selecting the location, consider the number of participants that you expect to attend the program, the teaching method, and accessibility. A unit-based program for a handful of people may be done in the break room, small conference room, or empty patient room. These locations should be easily accessible if staff have difficulty getting away from a clinical unit to attend an educational program. For a large group, you may want to select a conference room or an auditorium. The teaching method also influences your choice of location (Appendix F). An auditorium or large conference room is best for a lecture. A patient room or skill lab should be used if you are demonstrating equipment or practicing nursing skills.

7. How do I advertise a program?

A program offered internally may be advertised via word of mouth, e-mail, or eye-catching flyers posted in the work area. External programs may be advertised with professionally designed brochures or mailers. Whatever the method, advertising should provide information about the "who," "what," "when," "why," and "where" of the program. It should be interesting enough to catch a person's interest and explain "what's in it for me" so that people will want to attend (Appendices G and H).

8. Are there any general tips on preparing a flyer?

Program brochures and flyers should provide certain essential information such as the program title, date, start and end time, and location. Participants also want to know speaker name and program content and/or objectives. Additional information such as fees, refreshments, and need to preregister depends on your internal needs and processes. When designing flyers, use large type to make the title, date, and time stand out. Information about content, objectives, and other program details can be in a smaller type. Avoid using too many different type styles, all capital letters, or too much bold or underlining. These techniques can make the flyer more difficult to read. Arrange the information is short sentences or use bullets. A catchy title, interesting pictures, or use of different colored paper can make the information more noticeable. Finally, if you want an approximate count, ask participants to preregister.

9. How far in advance do I need to advertise a program?

A unit-based program should be advertised up to 2 weeks in advance. This schedule allows people who work part time, per diem, or on weekends to see the program notice and make plans to attend. A full-day seminar may be advertised up to 4 months in advance. This time frame allows participants to plan their schedules, arrange travel, and obtain conference funding.

10. How do I plan a program for nursing contact hours?

If nursing contact hours are to be awarded, a minimum of two RNs should participate in the planning. One person should be designated as the nurse planner with responsibility for the overall program delivery and coordination. People who are experts in the subject matter, representatives from the target audience, experts in education design, and speakers also should be included in the planning. Documentation that shows the use of the educational process is needed. This process is discussed in detail in Chapter 10.

11. What is involved in planning an all-day seminar?

Planning an all-day seminar can take considerable time and effort. A program planning committee should be organized so that the tasks can be divided. Planning begins 6 months to 1 year in advance. This time frame is needed particularly if you are booking national speakers and a banquet facility. Preparation, layout, and printing of a brochure also may take several weeks. Once organized, the planning committee needs to discuss the following: needs assessment, target audience, objectives, best teaching methods, time frames for each topic, speakers, location, budget and fees, refreshments, advertising, and need for contact hours. Sometimes it is helpful to use a checklist to make sure that all the details are covered, responsibility is assigned and a deadline date is set (see Appendix A).

12. How do I select a conference facility?

Set up a meeting with the banquet manager at the hotel or conference center so that you can tour the facility and discuss fees and services. Ask about room rental fees, cost of renting audiovisual equipment, catering, and any other charges. Also consider the following issues: How large or small a group can the site hold? Are breakout rooms available? How friendly and accommodating are the staff? Is nearby parking available? Is there a fee to park? Is the location easily accessible?

13. How do I determine budget and fees?

In planning a program, the following expenses should be considered: room rental, food, audiovisual equipment rental, speaker honoraria, speaker expenses, handouts, brochures, postage, and accreditation fees (Appendix I). These expenses may be covered by charging a fee to participants or seeking funding from a grant or company/corporate sponsorship (Appendix J). If funds are limited, costs can be cut by eliminating refreshments, seeking a location where there are no room rental costs, or considering cosponsorship with a company that can provide some financial support.

14. How do I decide what refreshments to offer?

A decision to provide refreshments is often based on the time and length of the program as well as funding. You may want to provide coffee, tea, and juice for a morning program. If funds allow, bagels, muffins, or doughnuts also may be served. A full-day program may or may not include lunch. If you choose not to provide lunch, be sure that easily accessible restaurants are available and that you have allowed adequate time for participants to eat lunch and return to the program. Refreshments for an afternoon break also should be considered: soda, pretzels, and cookies are possible choices. For a short (1- or 2-hour) program, it may not be necessary to offer refreshments. A program offered during the lunch or dinner hour may include a snack or beverage instead of a meal. If appropriate for the setting, you may even advise participants to bring their own snack, beverage, or lunch.

15. What are the different ways to set up a room for a training program?

A training room may be set up a number of different ways: classroom, theatre, dining room, meeting room, U-shaped style, or chevron style (see Appendix F). To be most effective, the teaching method and number of participants should govern the room set-up.

16. Is preregistration necessary?

Preregistration is recommended for several reasons. First it gives you an approximate count so that you will have enough handouts and refreshments. Second, if you will have more people than expected, you can prepare more handouts, add more chairs, adjust the room set-up or change the room location, or possibly close the registration to more participants. Finally, if registration numbers are low, you may consider canceling or readvertising the program.

17. Why may program registration be low?

Low program registration may be due to several factors. *Participants may not be aware of the program.* Evaluate to whom you sent your advertising and how you sent it. Did you send it to people who are most likely to be interested in attending? Did you use a method that is easily noticed (e.g., colorful flyers, eye-catching e-mail, high-visibility posting areas)?

Program time, length, or location can make attendance difficult. Is your program at a convenient time of day for participants? Some learners prefer to attend programs during the work day, whereas others do not. Some are just too busy to get away. Is program length (too long or too short) a factor? Is the location easily accessible to participants?

Participant interest also may be an issue. Evaluate how you determined the need for the program; be sure that you are offering a program that truly is needed. Make sure your advertising clearly outlines the importance of the program and how participants will benefit.

18. What should I be aware of if commercial support is provided for the program?

If you accept commercial support from a company for an educational program, it is important that the primary purpose is educational, not promotional. The program content should be objective and balanced, and monetary inducements beyond necessary expenses, gifts of more than nominal value, or personal amenities should be avoided.

If a commercial exhibit is to be part of the activity, it should not interfere with the presentation of the continuing education activity. Affiliations, sponsorships, financial support, and other potentially biasing factors should be disclosed to the audience (see Appendices E and J).

19. What are behavioral objectives?

Behavioral objectives are statements describing the behavior that the participant is expected to exhibit at the end of the learning experience. Well-written objectives are learner-oriented rather than content-oriented. Specifically, they describe the learner, include a statement of conditions, and identify the knowledge, skills, or feelings to be acquired. For example:

Learner	The orientee
Behavior	will demonstrate the correct procedure for endotracheal suctioning
Conditions	by the end of the class

20. How do I write objectives?

Writing behavioral objectives is more than an exercise in word-smithing. Ideally, they should communicate the intent and direction of the program. Behavioral objectives describe the learning experience and provide a framework for teaching-learning activities. They refer to the actions expected of the learner. For this reason, it is essential that the needs and abilities of the learner be considered in writing behavioral objectives.

Behavioral objectives are arranged into three groups: cognitive (knowledge), psychomotor (skills), and affective (feelings or values).

Cognitive objectives contain action verbs that describe knowledge. Verbs such as *recall, list, describe*, and *identify* are used: "By the end of the session, the participant will be able to recall the drugs that can be administered via an endotracheal tube during a code."

Psychomotor objectives contain verbs that describe motor skills. Verbs such as *imitates, demonstrates,* and *follows procedure* may be used: "By the end of the session, the participant will be able to demonstrate the correct procedure for endotracheal suctioning."

Affective objectives contain verbs that describe feelings or values. Verbs such as *shares, responds, defends,* and *acts consistently* may be used: (1) "During the session participants will share their most effective strategies for coping with stress." (2) "By the end of sensitivity training classes, the orientee will respond to the patient's needs for privacy in an appropriate manner."

21. Why are objectives necessary?

Because objectives describe the actions expected of the learner, they may be seen by some as a contract for what the participant will achieve by attending the program. From another perspective, they serve a promotional purpose and tell potential participants what the program is all about. Objectives also help determine the teaching method. Cognitive objectives may be met via a lecture, psychomotor objectives during a skill lab, and affective objectives during small group interactions.

Appendix A: Planning Committee/Program Coordinator Checklist

__ Select planning committee (2 RNs, one educator, members of target audience, subject matter experts)
__ Decide what specifically is needed and why (conduct/review your needs assessment data, determine topics)
__ Identify target audience
__ Formulate program goal and objectives
__ Decide on need for accreditation (contact hours) and select accrediting bodies (nursing only or others, such as medical education, social work)
__ Discuss the best teaching format for each topic and how the room should be set up
__ Decide time frame for each topic
__ Determine food, refreshments, and break times
__ Select training date and location; confirm and sign contract (if applicable)
__ Decide maximal/minimal number of participants
__ Discuss program budget (expenses, revenues)
__ Determine fee for program
__ Decide whether there will be vendors/displays and whether vendors will be charged a fee
__ Select speakers for each topic
__ Send speaker confirmation letters
__ Arrange audiovisual equipment (e.g., screen, microphones, slide projector, flipcharts, markers, overhead projector, laptop, LCD projector, TV/VCR, tape player, podium, laser pointer)
__ Design and distribute program advertising (flyers/brochure)

Up to 4 weeks before the program:
__ Complete contact hour paperwork for accreditation
__ Obtain handouts, biographical information from speakers
__ Arrange for speaker gifts, honorariums, travel, and lodging
__ Make copies, prepare participant handouts (don't forget an evaluation tool)
__ Confirm food, refreshments with training site and provide count
__ Confirm audiovisual equipment needed by speakers
__ Send confirmation letters to participants
__ Secure helpers for registration and audiovisual set-up, room monitors
__ Decide who will transport speakers to and from facility
__ Determine who will introduce speakers
__ Prepare welcome, introductory remarks
__ Prepare sign-in/registration lists
__ Prepare participant name tags

Day of the program: Arrive at least 1 hour before registration is to begin
__ Check room, refreshment set-up
__ Set up/test AV equipment
__ Prepare registration table (sign-in sheets, pens, handouts, name tags)
__ Greet speakers and review/set up AV equipment

Appendix B: Sample Confirmation Letter

February 21, 2002

Mary Smith
1234 Main Street
Anytown, USA 12345

Dear Mary:

Thank you for agreeing to present "Team Leadership, or How to be the Manager Everyone Wants to Work For" on Tuesday, May 23, from 8:30 AM to 12:00 noon at the First Presbyterian Church of the Covenant in Erie, Pa. As we discussed, Hamot will pay you a presentation honorarium of $___ plus $___ for your travel expenses.

My purchasing office has asked that you complete the enclosed W-9 form and return it to me. I will need this form submitted with the check request to process your honorarium. I will have a check available for you on the day of the presentation.

The program will be held at the First Presbyterian Church of the Covenant, located at 250 West 7th Street. I have enclosed a map and driving directions from Pittsburgh for you.

Your presentation will be part of our 2-day agenda. The program begins at 8:00 AM with a welcome and announcements. Your presentation is scheduled to begin at 8:30 am. The agenda is attached. We will have an overhead, VCR, and a wireless microphone in the room for you. If you need any other audiovisual equipment, please let me know. Please send me one copy of the handouts for your presentation by May 8 so that I can prepare the participant handouts.

I appreciate your willingness to present to our group. Please call me if you have any questions. My telephone number is ________________ and my e-mail address is ________________.

Sincerely,

Jean Bulmer, MSN, RNC
Manager, Center for Education & Staff Development

Appendix C: Sample Speaker Contract

Consultation/Speaking Agreement

This is an agreement between FACILITY NAME (hereafter referred to as FACILITY) and ____________________________________ (hereafter referred to as SPEAKER).

This agreement is for professional services to be rendered by SPEAKER on: __________ (date of program) to be held at __________________________ (location) from approximately _________ to ___________ (starting and ending time).

TERMS OF AGREEMENT

a. DESCRIPTION of services to be provided by SPEAKER:
(e.g., outline presentation times, topics)

b. FACILITY will arrange overnight accommodations for SPEAKER for the following date(s): ___________________. Accommodations will be for a standard room for one person. FACILITY will not be responsible for additional charges incurred during SPEAKER's stay (i.e., room service, additional guests, in-room movie rental, long-distance telephone calls, and other services).

c. Meals: FACILITY will reimburse or furnish meals for SPEAKER that would normally be eaten after arrival in (City) or prior to departure from (City). For example, if the SPEAKER arrives in (City) at 7 PM, no meals will be provided for that day. Meals that are reimbursed should be of reasonable cost: breakfast: $10; lunch, $15; dinner, $25. FACILITY will not be responsible for the meals of others traveling with the SPEAKER. FACILITY will provide the following meals on-site on the day of the program: (fill in meals to be provided/or if there is a meal that the speaker is to obtain at the hotel, such as breakfast).

d. Honorariums: FACILITY agrees to pay the SPEAKER $______ for the services described above.

e. Automobile travel: mileage/parking reimbursement: SPEAKER (*will/will not*) be reimbursed for parking fees while in (City) and (*will/will not*) be reimbursed for round-trip mileage between (City) and SPEAKER's home at the FACILITY standard mileage reimbursement rate of 32.5 cents per mile.

f. Air travel: FACILITY will arrange for air travel in coach class. FACILITY will reimburse for travel between hotel and airport terminals. Travel should be by the most appropriate method considering cost, availability, and time. Travel between hotel and FACILITY will be arranged by FACILITY.

g. FACILITY will be responsible for the conference room set-up, audiovisual equipment and other teaching aids, registration materials and handouts, awarding of contact hours, record keeping, and evaluations.

h. SPEAKER will submit receipts to FACILITY for reimbursable travel and food expenses as outlined above within 5 days after presentation.

i. SPEAKER will advise FACILITY in the development of presentation objectives, content, and program advertising. SPEAKER will submit audiovisual equipment needs and room set-up needs to FACILITY at least 2 weeks prior to the presentation. SPEAKER will provide one copy of participant handouts for FACILITY to duplicate for program participants at least 2 weeks prior to presentation.

j. Cancellation of agreement: FACILITY may cancel this agreement without penalty up to 7 days prior to the date of the presentation if there is insufficient preregistration.

(List any other reasons if applicable.)

Signatures:

______________________________	______________________________
SPEAKER	FACILITY
______________________________	______________________________
DATE	DATE

Appendix D: Sample Speaker Information Form

This form can be given to the speaker so that he or she is familiar with your program and target audience.

Program title ______________________________

Date ____________________ Time ____________________

Location (name, address, room) ______________________________

How the need for the program was identified ______________________________

____

Purpose/theme of the program ______________________________

Target audience ______________________________

Speaker's topic ______________________________

Start and end time ______________________________

Key objectives ______________________________

____

____

Key issues/topics that we would like the speaker to address ______________________________

____

Other speakers' names and topics

____

____

____

How room will be set up ______________________________

Audience information

Sensitive issues affecting the group, organization or industry ______________________________

____

Number attending ____________________ Age ranges ____________________

Appendix E: Sample Disclosure Form

FACULTY DISCLOSURE OF COMMERCIAL SUPPORT

Name: ______________________________

Presentation topic: ______________________________

Date presented: ______________________________

Your willingness to take the time to prepare and present an educational program is greatly appreciated. As a sponsor of nursing continuing education activities, (FACILITY NAME) requests disclosure to the audience of the existence of any relationship between a faculty member/their department and a commercial company. This relationship may be in the form of support for your presentation or related to the content of your presentation. The existence of a relationship does not imply anything improper, nor does it decrease the value of your presentation. Please detail any financial arrangements or affiliations with any corporate organization which may pose a real or apparent conflict of interest.

Affiliation/Financial Interest	**Name of Corporation**
Grants/research support	____________________
Consultant	____________________
Speaker's bureau	____________________
Major stock shareholder	____________________
Other financial or material interest	____________________

____________________ ____________________

Signature Date

Appendix F: Room Set-up Styles

Classroom style
Consists of tables and chairs arranged in rows. Can be used for small or large groups. Table provides a place for writing and materials.

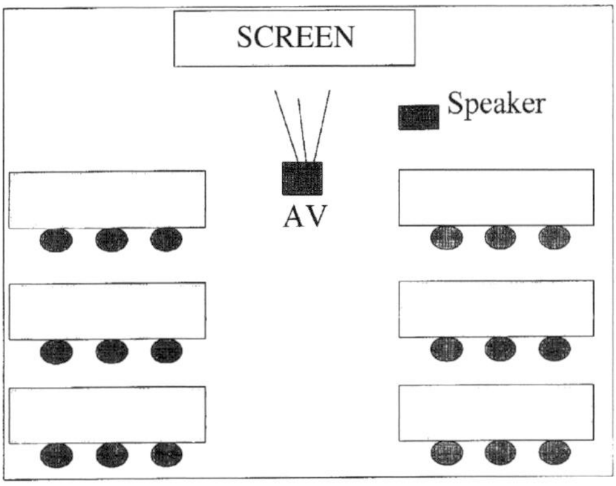

Lecture, auditorium, or theater style
Consists of chairs arranged in rows or a semicircle shape. Normally used for large groups or when space is limited. Lack of a writing surface and the closeness of the chairs can be a problem.

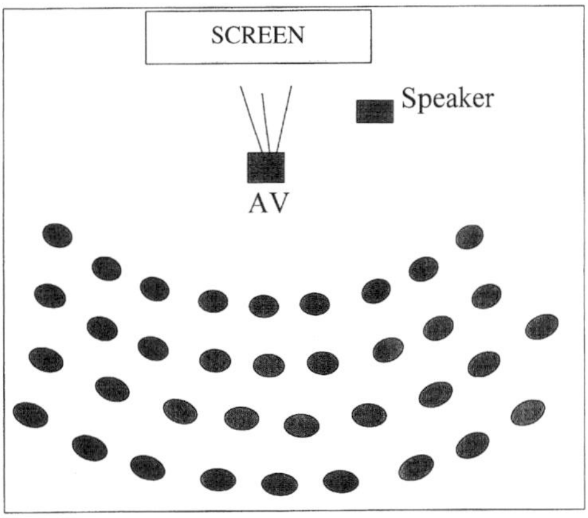

Dining style
An informal style, may be used in a banquet facility. Tables are set with seats on one half only. Sometimes half-round tables may be provided. Allows seating of large groups with small group interaction at the tables. Allows the speaker to wander between tables to interact with participants.

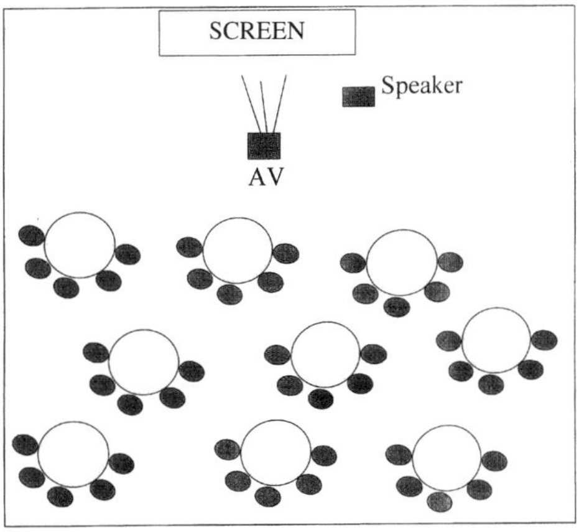

Meeting or conference style
Seats are arranged around a conference room table. Depending on table size, this style can accommodate 12 or more participants. Design allows participants to interact easily with each other.

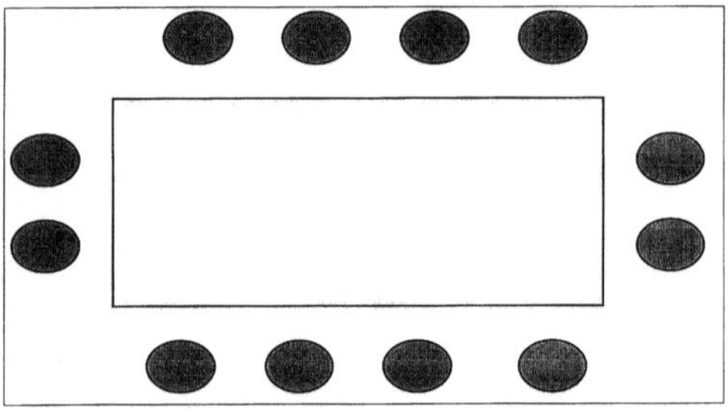

U-shaped style
Seats are arranged in a U shape. Design allows participants to interact easily with each other as well as view a formal presentation.

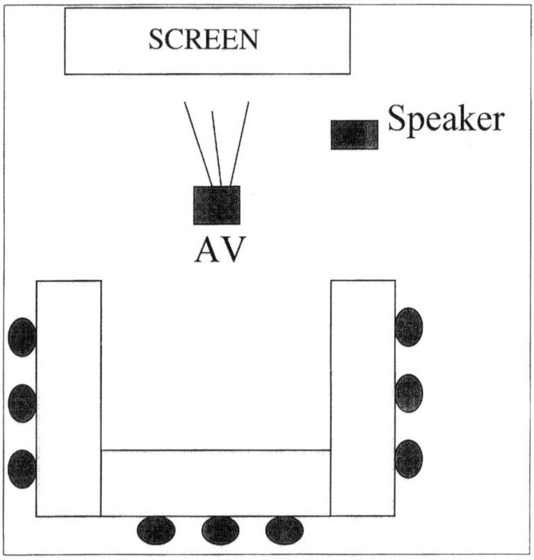

Chevron style
A variation of the classroom style. The angle of the tables allows participants to see each other on each side of the room; hence, this design allows more interaction between participants than the classroom style.

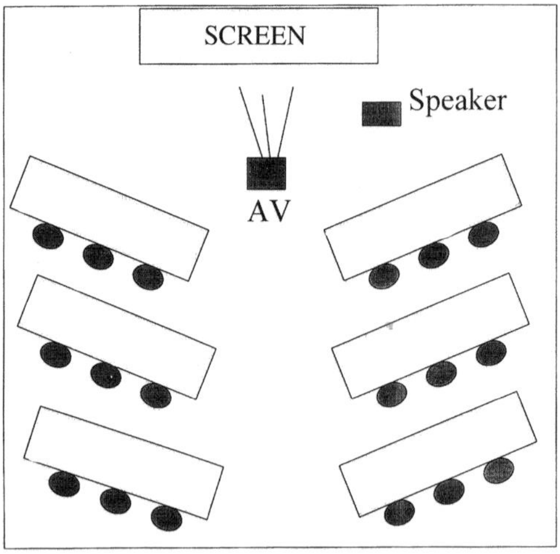

Appendix G: Single-page flyer

Understanding & Supervising the Twenty-Somethings

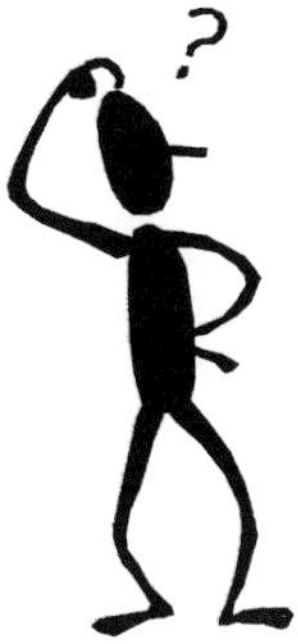

Thursday, September 30, 1999

12:00 pm – 1:00 pm

G3 conference room

presented by Jean Bulmer

They are sometimes referred to as Generation X, Baby Busters, or YIFFIES. Who are these people? What are their motivators and defining characteristics? What factors have molded their approach to life? Which techniques are useful in supervising and managing this newest member of the adult workforce?

This one hour session will:

- Highlight the societal factors that influenced the development of "Generation Xers"
- Review common myths and misconceptions of this generation
- Outline the motivators, desires and needs of the Twenty-Somethings

Advance registration is requested in order to ensure adequate seating, beverages, and handouts. Pop will be provided. Please bring your lunch. To register, call the Center for Education voice mail registration line at x 4265.

Appendix H: Trifold flyer (2 pages)

CRIES Pain Assessment
Infant I.V. Workshop
Wednesday, May 30, 2001

Educational Credit

Hamot Medical Center Nursing Continuing Education Provider Unit is accredited as a provider of continuing education in nursing by the American Nurses Credentialing Center's Commission on Accreditation. Participants will be awarded 3.9 contact hours. *Please note: you must attend the entire session in order to receive credit.*

Program Information

For questions and/or information please call Hamot Medical Center, Neonatal Intensive Care Unit at — — —. If you are in need of an accommodation, due to disability, to participate in this program, we ask that we receive this notification one week before the program so that we may make the necessary arrangements.

Speakers

Nell Nipper, RNC, is a CN-IVA in the Neonatal Intensive Care Unit at Hamot Medical Center. She has over 25 years experience as a caregiver in the NICU.

Margaret McGraw, BSN, RNC, is a CN-IVB in the Neonatal Intensive Care Unit at Hamot Medical Center. She has 18 years experience as a caregiver in the NICU and 15 years experience as a NICU Transport Nurse.

Directions to Hamot

Hamot Medical Center is located on State Street in downtown Erie, two blocks south of Presque Isle Bay. To reach Hamot from Interstate 79, follow the Bayfront Highway about three miles to State Street. Turn right on State Street. Hamot will be on your left. A parking garage is located on 3rd Street between State Street and French, and surface parking lot (parking meters) at 2nd and French Streets.

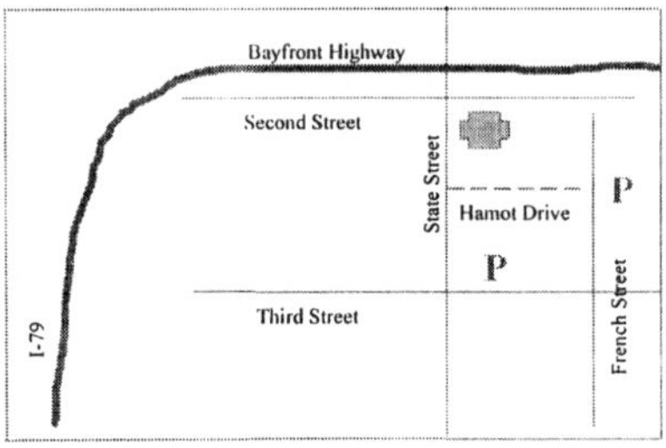

CRIES Pain Assessment
Infant I.V. Workshop

Wednesday, May 30, 2001

at

Hamot Medical Center

Choice of 3 sessions: 8 am, noon, or 4 pm

Hamot Health Foundation's Neonatal Intensive Care Unit Presents:

CRIES Pain Assessment
Infant I.V. Workshop

Wednesday, May 30, 2001

Choice of 3 Sessions:

8 am – 11:30 am
12 noon – 3:30 pm
4 pm – 7:30 pm

at
Hamot Medical Center
Ground Floor Conference Room
201 State Street
Erie, PA 16550

Program Goal: Provide information on Neonatal and Pediatric issues, specifically pain assessment and I.V. therapy

Program Content: Review of CRIES Neonatal/Infant Pain Assessment Scale
Discussion of Neonatal and Pediatric Peripheral I.V. Therapy
Equipment and its uses (T-connectors, IV caths, pumps)
Practice session on life-life models (scalp, arm, leg)

Class Size: Each sessions is limited to 20 participants.

Course Fee/Registration: $20 fee includes bag lunch or dinner, program, and contact hours. The registration deadline is May 23, 2001. Cancellation policy: one week notice is required to receive a full refund.

☆☆☆☆☆☆☆☆☆☆☆☆☆☆☆☆☆☆☆☆☆☆☆☆☆☆☆☆☆☆☆☆☆☆☆☆☆☆

CRIES Pain Assessment ❖ Infant I.V. Workshop Registration Form

Name: ______________________________ Employer ______________________________

Address: ____
number & street city, state, & zip

Register me for the following session (check only one):
_____ 8 am – 11.30 am _____ 12 noon –3:30 pm _____ 4 pm – 7:30 pm

$20 fee includes bag lunch or dinner, program, and contact hours. Please make checks payable to Hamot Medical Center. Send registration and fee to: Susan Rodgers, RNC, Unit Nurse Manager, Neonatal Intensive Care Unit, Hamot Medical Center, 201 State Street, Erie, PA 16550.

Appendix I: Budget/Fees

Below is a list of possible program expenses. Specific items will not be applicable in every case:
• Room rental
• Food, refreshments, tax, gratuity, set-up charge
• Audiovisual equipment rental
• Speaker honorariums
• Other speaker expenses: travel (airfare, car rental, mileage, taxi), food, lodging
• Handouts: copying, binding, paper
• Brochures, flyers: layout, printing/copying, folding, paper, mailing label lists, postage
• Name tags, receipt books
• Contact hour/accreditation fees
• Room decorations (banners, flowers)
• Speaker gifts, door prizes
Possible revenue sources:
• Charge participants a fee
• Invite company/corporate sponsorship
• Invite vendors to have a display table and charge a fee
• Cosponsor program with another company that can provide some funds

Appendix J: Sample Commercial Support Agreement

FACILITY NAME (hereafter referred to as FACILITY) agrees to accept commercial support from ____________________________ in the amount of ____________ for the continuing education activity ____________________ to be held at __________ on ________________.

This is: ☐ an unrestricted educational grant
☐ a designated grant for ____________________________
(Travel Only, Honorarium Only, Support for catering functions, equipment loan, brochure distribution, etc.)

Both parties agree that:

1. The program will be conducted for the purpose of the education of the audience and for the benefit of the health care consumer. Its primary purpose is not for the benefit of the commercial supporters, providers, or presenters involved in the activity (educational, not promotional).
2. The program will be objective and, when legitimate differences or contrasting views exist, balanced.
3. Factors that can result in the introduction of bias will be avoided. These may include monetary inducements beyond necessary expenses, gifts of more than nominal value, or personal amenities.
4. The design and production of continuing nursing educational activities shall be the responsibility of the FACILITY. This responsibility includes selection/approval of topics, presenters, educational materials, and the administration of the activities. The FACILITY will ensure that the design, presenters and materials are free of endorsement and bias.
5. Affiliations, sponsorships, financial support and other potentially biasing factors will be disclosed to the audience.
6. If a commercial exhibit is to be part of the activity, it will not influence planning or interfere with the presentation of the continuing education activity. When possible, exhibits and promotional materials will not be displayed or distributed in the same room as the educational activity. If this is not possible, there will be some method of separating the exhibits from part of the room used for educational presentation.
7. Representatives of the commercial supporter may attend the educational activities as long as the representatives do not engage in sales or promotional activities while the educational presentation is taking place.
8. The FACILITY will be responsible for and accountable for the administration of the financial aspects of the educational activity.

9. Following the CNE activity, upon request, the FACILITY will send a report to each commercial supporter detailing the expenditure of funds each has provided. Each commercial supporter will report information to the FACILITY concerning their expenditures in support of the activity.

______________________	______________________
FACILITY	COMMERCIAL SUPPORT PROVIDER
______________________	______________________
DATE	DATE

BIBLIOGRAPHY

1. Bice-Stephens W: Designing a conference—from start to finish. J Cont Educ Nurs 32:198–202, 2001.
2. Brady M: So you want to host a nursing conference? J Cont Educ Nurs 27:89–94, 1996.
3. Waddell DL, Hummel ME: Systematic planning of continuing nursing education. J Nurses Staff Dev 15: 163–166, 1999.

10. CREDENTIALING

Jean M. Bulmer, MSN, RNC

1. What are CEUs, CERPS, clock hours, credit hours, and contact hours?

They are units of educational measurement used by various accrediting bodies. CEU is the acronym for continuing education unit; CERP refers to continuing education recognition program. These terms describe the amount of time awarded to participants in an educational program.

2. What does it mean when someone asks if a program is accredited, or has credits, CEUs, or contact hours?

An educational program may be accredited or have credits, CEUs, or contact hours if it has undergone a process to ensure that it meets certain educational standards. The process for accreditation and the specific requirements are determined by an accrediting body. For nursing, the accrediting body is the American Nurses Credentialing Center, Commission on Accreditation. Many disciplines have their own accrediting body. The table below lists the various accrediting bodies. Although many people use the terms *credits, CEUs,* and *contact hours* interchangeably, the correct term for referring to the nursing hours awarded by the American Nurses Credentialing Center is contact hours.

DISCIPLINE	ACCREDITING BODY
Medicine	Accreditation Council for Continuing Medical Education
Psychology	American Psychological Association, Committee on Accreditation
Social work	Council on Social Work Education
Intravenous therapy	Intravenous Nurses Certification Corporation
Oncology nursing, pediatric oncology, advanced oncology	Oncology Nursing Certification Corporation
Physical therapy, occupational therapy	Executive Council of Physical Therapy and Occupational Therapy Examiners
Adult day services, assisted living, behavioral health, employment and community services, medical rehabilitation	Commission on Accreditation and Rehabilitation Facilities

3. My employer awards certificates of attendance. How are they different?

Some employers prepare certificates of attendance for some or all of their programs so that the participants can have a personal record of their attendance. These programs may or may not meet the definition of continuing education. Certificates of attendance often include the program name, date, location, and duration. The certificate does not have an accreditation statement. In some cases, the certificate can serve as a record of participation for people who need to submit continuing education hours. Each accrediting body establishes guidelines for accreditation, including the acceptance of nonaccredited education hours.

4. Can all programs be accredited for contact hours?

Contact hour accreditation can be awarded only for programs that meet the definition of continuing education. The program must go beyond basic knowledge, enhance the person's practice, and be applicable beyond a specific work setting. Contact hours are not awarded for orientation and basic education programs.

5. What is joint sponsorship?

Two or more groups may work together to plan an educational program. These groups may be hospitals or even include two or more disciplines. When joint sponsorship is planned, it is wise to have a written agreement that details the financial and logistical responsibilities of each party.

6. Is joint sponsorship a good or bad idea?

Joint sponsorship can be beneficial, especially if the groups have limited resources that can be maximized by working together. One important point is that each group will be focused on the needs of its constituents. Medical education focuses on ensuring that the program meets the accreditation standards for physicians and that the education needs of physicians are met. Nursing education takes a similar stance from a nursing perspective.

7. How are contact hours calculated?

Fifty minutes of organized educational activity equals 1 contact hour. Time spent on welcome, introductions, breaks, and viewing of exhibits is not included in the calculation of contact hours. An easy way to calculate the contact hours is to total the number of minutes in the program and then divide by 50. For example, a 2-hour program is 120 minutes long:

$$120 \div 50 = 2.4$$

The program is awarded 2.4 contact hours.

8. Why are contact hours needed?

Nurses who hold a specialty certification require continuing education hours to maintain their certification. In addition, a number of states require continuing education hours for licensure and relicensure (see Chapter 20).

9. A staff member renewing her certification lost her contact hour certificates. Can they be reissued?

Accrediting agencies are required to keep attendance records for 5 years. The staff member can contact the agency that awarded the contact hours and request another certificate. She may need to provide program titles and dates because attendance must be verified by checking attendance records.

10. Can nursing contact hours be awarded to non-nurses?

Yes. There are no restrictions placed on who may be awarded a nursing contact hour certificate. Some non-nursing professional associations accept nursing contact hours for their constituents. Non-nurses should be advised to contact their professional organization for details.

11. What is the process for obtaining contact hours for an educational program?

Contact hours can be obtained by submitting program information to a contact hour approver or by working with a contact hour provider. Specific information that is needed includes needs assessment, goals, objectives, content, teaching methods, target audience, faculty qualifications, description of the physical facilities, and an evaluation tool.

12. What is the difference between an approver and a provider?

Agencies that are **approvers** of continuing education in nursing review educational activities developed by others verify that the activity meets certain criteria and award contact hours. Many state nurses associations, federal nursing services, and specialty nursing organizations are approvers. Agencies that are **providers** of continuing education in nursing develop and provide their own educational activities and ensure that they meet certain criteria in order to award contact hours. Providers may be any organization responsible for the overall development, implementation, evaluation, and quality assurance of continuing education in nursing. Providers are permitted to work with nonaccredited organizations seeking continuing education credit for an educational activity. This practice is called coproviding.

13. Who awards approver and provider status?

Accredited approver and accredited provider status are awarded by the American Nurses Credentialing Center's Commission on Accreditation. Accredited approvers also may award approved provider status (see table on following page).

14. Describe the process for becoming an approver or provider.

Applicants for approver status must submit applications to the American Nurses Credentialing Center's Commission on Accreditation. Those seeking provider status can submit applications either to the American Nurses Credentialing Center's Commission on Accreditation or to an accredited approver.

15. What material is submitted in the application to become an approver or provider?

The application includes organizational charts, an explanation of education processes, and samples of educational programs that have been offered by the applicant. Applications are reviewed by peer reviewers, and a site visit may be conducted to verify, clarify, and amplify the information contained in the application.

16. Why seek accreditation?

Accreditation is a voluntary process that recognizes the quality of an individual activity and the provider.

17. Why are the accreditation statements so long?

Accreditation statements are intended to describe accurately the accrediting body. They tell whether the program is accredited by an accredited provider, an accredited approver, or an approved provider (see table on following page).

18. What are disclosure statements? Why are they needed?

Disclosure statements are used to advise the participants of any relationship between a faculty member or department and a commercial company. This relationship may be in the form of support for the presentation or may be related to the content of their presentation. Disclosure of the relationship does not imply anything improper, nor does it decrease the value of a presentation. It simply alerts the audience that a relationship exists. Presenters are expected to present an unbiased view.

19. Can credit be awarded for independent study?

Video, print, and computer instruction are forms of independent study and continuing education for which contact hours can be awarded. The activities must be designed so that there is a way to measure achievement of objectives and provide feedback to the learner about successful completion.

20. I offered a program last week, and now the staff are asking if they can get contact hour credit. Can they?

No. The accreditation standards require that the credit designation must be awarded before the program occurs. It is the responsibility of the provider or approver to ensure that the program meets the accreditation criteria, communicate that it is accredited, and detail the requirements for successful completion in advance. You can award an internal certificate of attendance instead.

21. I want to submit a continuing education application for an upcoming program. What do I need to do?

First, contact your local approver body (e.g., state nurses association) and request an application for program approval. The application should have detailed instructions about what must be submitted for approval. Typically, you must have a planning committee that includes a registered nurse and others who represent the target audience and have content expertise. You must document why the program is needed and how it will enhance the nurses' practice. You need to submit biographical

Types of Nursing Accreditation Designated by the American Nurses Credentialing Center's Commission on Accreditation

TYPE OF ACCREDITATION	ACCREDITED APPROVER	ACCREDITED PROVIDER	APPROVED PROVIDER	CONTACT HOUR CREDIT FOR PROGRAMS
Who may apply	State nurses associations, federal nursing services, and specialty nursing organizations	Any organization responsible for overall development, implementation, evaluation, and quality of continuing education in nursing	Any organization responsible for overall development, implementation, evaluation, and quality of continuing education in nursing	Any group responsible for development, implementation, and evaluation of a nursing continuing education activity
Reviewing body	American Nurses Credentialing Center's Commission on Accreditation	American Nurses Credentialing Center's Commission on Accreditation	Accredited approver	Accredited approver
Fee	$3500–4500 + site visit expenses	$3500–4500 + site visit expenses	Varies	Varies
Site visit	Required	Required	No	No
Role/activities	Review educational activities developed by others and award contact hours *and* designate approver status to organizations responsible for continuing education in nursing	Develop and award contact hours for their own educational activities	Develop and award contact hours for their own educational activities	Planning committee prepares an application to seek credit for a single program
Credit statement	(Approver name) is accredited as an approver of continuing nursing education by the American Nurses Credentialing Center's Commission on Accreditation	(Provider name) is accredited as a provider of continuing nursing education by the American Nurses Credentialing Center's Commission on Accreditation	(Provider name) is approved as a provider of continuing nursing education by (approver name), which is accredited as an approver of continuing nursing education by the American Nurses Credentialing Center's Commission on Accreditation	This program is approved for x contact hours by the (approver name), which is accredited as an approver of continuing nursing education by the American Nurses Credentialing Center's Commission on Accreditation
Accreditation term	6 yr	6 yr	2 yr	2 yr

information about the presenters that establishes their qualification to present on the selected topics. A form describing the program's behavioral objectives, content, time frames, and teaching methods is also needed, along with an evaluation form that asks specific questions about the effectiveness of the program. Once your application is complete, it is sent to the approver for review. There is a fee for approval, and the amounts are set by the approver. Applications should be submitted as far in advance as possible. Submission time frames may require you to submit the application many weeks in advance to allow adequate time for review. Approved programs are accredited for a 2-year term and can be offered as many times as you like during that period.

BIBLIOGRAPHY

1. American Nurses Credentialing Center's Commission on Accreditation: Manual for Accreditation as a Provider of Continuing Nursing Education. Washington, DC, American Nurses Credentialing Center, 2000–2001.
2. American Nurses Credentialing Center On-line: www.nursingworld.orc/ancc.

11. WHEN THE PROBLEM IS NOT AN EDUCATIONAL ISSUE

Sandra L. Spangenberg, RN, BSN

1. Are all requests for education truly educational needs?

No. Educational needs are identified based on performance problems or discrepancies between actual and desired performance. Performance problems caused by a lack of knowledge, skills, or attitudes may be resolved with education, but not all performance problems are due to these deficits. Performance problems also may be caused by other issues. For example, after an increase in falls, the manager of the medical-surgical unit requests education in the proper use of gait belts. As you follow up on the request, you find that there has been a shortage of gait belts. When gait belts are available, staff use them correctly. No amount of education will resolve the problem. This example illustrates the importance of evaluating all requests for education and not assuming that education will resolve each performance problem. To plan useful educational offerings, it is essential that the educator differentiate between educational and noneducational performance problems.

2. What are the potential causes of noneducational performance problems?

There are numerous causes of performance problems that cannot be resolved by education. The previous example described a performance problem related to a shortage of supplies. Other issues that the educator may consider in evaluating performance problems include the following:

- Inadequate staffing. Are staff members unable to perform because they are short of help or working extra shifts, which causes an increase in errors and short cuts?
- Malfunctioning equipment. Are mistakes due to equipment error?
- Lack of guidelines for performance. Are unclear policies and procedures causing inconsistency in performance?
- Unrealistic expectations. Are staff members expected to perform beyond their scope of practice?

Education will not affect performance problems related to these issues. A necessary step in the education planning process is to verify the existence of an educational need.

3. Why is it so important to differentiate between educational and noneducational performance problems?

The current health care economy has led to decreased budgets and downsized departments. Staff development departments must demonstrate their value by focusing efforts on meeting educational needs. Planning education that teaches what is already known wastes the educator's and learner's time and the organization's dollars. Education that is valued is linked to desired performance as well as the organization's mission and objectives. Educators who take these issues into consideration increase their value within the organization.

4. How can I analyze performance problems to identify educational issues?

To analyze a performance problem, you should ask two questions:

1. Does the employee know what is expected?
2. Does the employee have the skills and competencies to meet these expectations?

If the answer to both questions is yes, the performance problem is not educational. The employee has the knowledge and skills to perform, and education will not change performance. If the answer to either question is no, a deficit in knowledge or skills has been identified. Education will be a good investment of the educator's, learner's, and organization's time and efforts.

5. How can I determine the cause of performance problems that are not related to educational needs?

A series of questions can be asked to determine the cause of performance problems that are not educational. If the employee has the skills but is not demonstrating them, ask why. Are there barriers to performing according to standards, such as inadequate supplies or staff?

Examine the consequences of performing correctly or incorrectly. If the nursing assistant (NA) who completes an assignment in a timely manner receives additional work, will he or she continue to work as efficiently? If the RN who socializes and does not complete an assignment on time gets a decreased patient load, is there a reason to stop socializing? Evaluating consequences can help the educator identify reasons for nonperformance. If the employee is simply refusing to demonstrate skills and meet performance expectations, it is an accountability issue, and the coaching-discipline process begins.

6. Is evaluation really part of my role as an educator? Shouldn't managers evaluate their employees' performance?

Yes, performance evaluation is a function of the manager's role. However, educators are well versed in evaluating competency and problem solving and can assist the manager in identifying the causes of performance problems. As partners in this process, you and the nurse manger can identify performance problems, determine causes, and strategize to resolve them. This team focus further demonstrates an educator's worth in the organization.

7. What can I do to assist a manger in understanding when the problem is not an educational need?

As in all working relationships, communication is essential. Developing a partnership approach to resolving performance problems can lead to successful outcomes. Initially, you and the managers with whom you deal can work together to determine individual responsibilities in resolving performance problems. Often the educator must educate the manager about the process used to identify and resolve problems. A nonthreatening approach with focus on the improvements in patient outcomes can be helpful.

Together you and the manager can ask the questions that determine the cause of performance problems. When the cause is lack of knowledge, skills, or attitude, you should take the primary responsibility. Education is planned with the manager's input into desired outcomes. When performance problems are due to systemic issues, you can assist in their resolution by facilitating interdisciplinary problem solving, developing policies and procedures, or resolving other process issues. When an accountability issue is identified, the manager takes the primary role. Your expertise in developing objectives can assist in goal setting throughout the disciplinary process. You also can assist in coaching the employee to improve performance.

8. What is coaching?

Coaching is an effective tool in resolving performance problems. As a coach, you can help employees reach their full potential and develop as a valuable member of the team. To be effective, the core principles of coaching must be considered:

- Focusing on improvement of job performance rather than changing personality
- Respecting the dignity and worth of the individual employee
- Focusing on the current level of performance

9. How can I coach employees to improve performance?

To achieve the successful outcomes as a coach, follow these steps:

1. *Analyze the performance concern before meeting with the employee.* Review the facts; do not base your analysis on rumors or hearsay, which often are unreliable. Determine the importance of the concern: is it significant or annoying? Is there value in changing performance?

2. *Establish a climate for positive rapport.* Coaching is done in private. It is a one-on-one conversation. The educator must show concern for the employee.

3. *Help the employee recognize that a concern exists.* Calmly identify the performance problem and explain why it is a concern. These are your concerns—not what someone else has said. Again, discuss behavior instead of personal traits. Share specific and objective accounts of actual performance. Avoid judgement words such as *good, bad,* or *should.*

4. *Ask for the employee's perspective.* Listen empathetically. Paraphrase the employee's version to be certain that you have a good understanding.

5. *Involve the employee in solving the problem.* Ask the employee to generate solutions. Provide input into the solutions. Be careful of giving unsolicited advice. Ultimately the employee needs to own the solution.

6. *Mutually agree on the actions to be taken and the follow-up.* The educator as well as the employee is a part of the plan. Identify obstacles that you will clear. Be available for support and questions. Set timelines for improvement. End on a positive note. Demonstrate confidence that the behavior can be improved.

7. *Follow up.* Evaluate progress together. Provide feedback that focuses on behavior instead of personal traits. Meaningful feedback should be given immediately. Avoid time lapses between performance and feedback.

8. Finally, *congratulate each other on progress.*

10. How can coaching work in everyday situations?

The steps of coaching outlined above are exemplified in the following narrative:

A nurse new to the critical care unit was admitting a patient with extremely high blood pressure. The admitting orders included Nipride for the elevated blood pressure. The preceptor watched as the orientee took vital signs, determined that the blood pressure was elevated, and continued to complete the database.

1. After seeing that the orientee was not going to start the Nipride, the preceptor took over, saying, "I'm going to help you. Let's work together." When the crisis was resolved, the preceptor saw that the orientee was visibly shaken. She decided that they needed time to review the experience.

2. The preceptor asked another nurse to cover and said, "Come on, let's get a soda at the cafeteria."

3. After they sat down the preceptor said, "You know that patient's blood pressure was dangerously high, and since we had an order for Nipride, it needed to be our first priority."

4. The preceptor allowed the orientee to talk. The nurse said, "Oh, I knew that I needed to do something about the blood pressure, but when I thought about the Nipride, I kept thinking, how do I set it up? What will the drip rate be? And I just got flustered."

5. The preceptor responded, "Well, I can understand that it's scary, but we'll have to do something. Do you have any ideas?" The orientee answered, "Well, I can make a cheat sheet with the drug dosages and keep it with me."

6. "Good idea," said the preceptor. "And the next time that a patient with elevated blood pressure is admitted, you can take it. Let's look at this as a learning experience. I'm glad that we talked." "I am, too," said the orientee.

7. The orientee was assigned a patient with elevated blood pressure at a later date. With the preceptor's guidance she successfully managed the patient's care. Both reviewed the difference between the two episodes and felt positive about the orientee's success.

8. After the successful management they went to the cafeteria again—this time to celebrate their success.

BIBLIOGRAPHY

1. Alspach JG: The Educational Process in Nursing Staff Development. St. Louis, Mosby, 1995.
2. Jerome PJ: Coaching Through Effective Feedback: A Practical Guide to Successful Communication. Irvine, CA, Richard Chang Associates, 1994.
3. Mager RF, Pipe P: Analyzing Performance Problems or You Really Oughta Wanna. Belmont, CA, Lake Publishing, 1997.
4. Puetz BE: Needs assessment: The essence of staff development programs. In Kelly KJ: Nursing Staff Development: Current Competence, Future Focus. Philadelphia, J.B. Lippincott, 1992, pp 97–116.

III. *Creating a Learning Environment*

12. ADULT LEARNING THEORY

Daryl Boucher, RN, MSN, EMT-P

1. What is adult learning theory'?

Adult learning theory is a set of principles and philosophies guiding the instruction of adults. The best known of these learning theories is **andragogy**, the art and science of helping adults learn.[6] The term is associated with a particular approach to the education of adults and is based on the appreciation and recognition that adults learn differently from children, have a different motivation for learning, and possess valuable life experience that can augment learning. Andragogic principles are an organized effort to help adults function as self-directed, life-long learners.

2. Why should I be interested in learning about andragogy?

As an educator of adults, you teach people with a wide range of skills, knowledge, experience, and abilities. Knowledge of adult learning theory helps you understand how and why learning occurs. In addition, the andragogic principles provide an excellent framework for classroom management and outline the role and characteristics of both students and instructor.

3. Until recently I had not heard of adult learning theory. Why the sudden interest?

Educators are realizing that adults do learn differently from children. Adults also have expectations that the programs that they attend will be of high quality. Staff development professionals need to utilize novel, creative, cost-effective ways of delivering education to adults.

Moreover, rapid technologic advances and the knowledge explosion of this century have had and will continue to have a dramatic effect on the health care setting. The renewed emphasis on adult learning theory is a reflection of the rapid explosion of knowledge. It is estimated that the half-life of medical and nursing knowledge is approximately five years. In other words, five years after graduating from a formal education program, one-half of what was learned is obsolete. Clearly, there has never been a time in the history of health care when lifelong learning has been so crucial. More adults are finding themselves back in the classroom at work. New procedures, evidence-based learning, scientific advances, and development of new medications demand ongoing education. In addition, health care delivery is constantly changing, driven in large part by the payer systems. The health care structure has become focused on outcomes. To be accountable, staff educators must be able to demonstrate that what they present in the classroom has a positive effect on patient outcomes.

4. What are the concepts of adult learning theory?

Malcolm Knowles is often cited as the father of andragogy, although many other behavioralists, humanists, sociologists, psychologists, educators, and developmentalists have contributed to the concepts. The essential principles of andragogy can be summarized as follows:

1. Adults desire and enact a tendency toward self-directedness, although they may be dependent in some situations. As people mature, their self-concept moves from dependent personalities toward self-directing adults who know what they want, when they want it.

2. Adults accumulate a greater volume and different quality of experience throughout their lifetime, especially in comparison with younger learners. This experience is a rich resource for learning; personal experiences establish self-identity and are highly valued. Adults also learn better from experiential teaching methods.

3. Adults' readiness to learn becomes increasingly related to the developmental tasks of their social roles. Readiness to learn peaks when adults assume new life roles (e.g., new job, parenthood) or when they experience a need to know in order to perform more effectively in some aspect of their lives.

4. Adults are competency-based, performance-centered learners. As people mature, their time perspective changes from postponed application of knowledge to immediate application; adults want to be able to use and apply what they learn. Their orientation is task- or problem-centered. Adults want to learn in order to solve immediate problems.

5. All adults are motivated to learn. However, the more potent motivators are internal: self-esteem, recognition, better quality of life, and greater self-confidence.

5. What are the characteristics of adult learners?

Although clearly not every learner is the same, adults possess many similar characteristics that are important for the educator to recognize. Characteristics of adult learners, in addition to the assumptions described above, include the following:

- Readiness to learn depends on previous learning.
- Intrinsic motivation produces more pervasive and permanent learning.
- More and different types of life experiences are organized differently from those of children.
- Adults prefer different types of personal learning style.
- Adults desire to be connected and supported by one another; they appreciate the option of group work but also can work independently.
- Individual responsibilities and life situations provide a social context that affects learning.
- Adults appreciate information that is presented in an organized, logical manner.
- Learning is enhanced by repetition.
- Adults learn at different rates.
- Adults learn by doing.
- Adults want feedback and opportunities for practice.
- Adults want to participate as "partners" in the learning process.
- Adults recognize the need to participate in lifelong learning activities.
- The ability to learn is maintained throughout life.
- A gradual decline in physical and sensory capabilities may affect motivation and teaching methods.

Principles that facilitate adult learning include the following:

- The learning is voluntary and self-initiated.
- The learning is self-controlled and self-directed.
- The learning is related to an immediate need, problem, or identified deficit.
- The teacher assumes the role of facilitator.
- Information and assignments are viewed as pertinent.
- New material should draw on past experiences.
- The threat to self is reduced to a minimum.
- The nature of the learning activity changes frequently.
- The teacher demonstrates mutual respect for the student.
- The student is an active contributor and vested partner in the learning situation.
- The environment is conducive to learning.
- The environment is free from distractions and is comfortable.

6. How difficult is it for a nurse educator to apply the principles of adult learning theory?

The same concepts that nurses use when teaching patients will assist staff educators when teaching nurses:

- Encourage learners' identification of their own learning needs.
- Encourage learners to outline personal goals.
- Collaborate to accomplish goals.
- Encourage the learner's independence, self-direction, and autonomy.

- Value individual differences and the need to develop mutual trust and respect.
- Evaluate shared responsibility for the accomplishment of goals.

Keeping these concepts in mind, nurse educators will find it easier to incorporate the principles of adult learning into their training.

7. I teach mandatory inservices for my organization. How can I help people to learn when they do not appear to be interested in the particular topic?

This problem is one of the greatest challenges for staff educators. Motivation is at the core of why people behave as they do. *The main influence on learning and motivation is the participants themselves.* However, the staff educator can employ certain strategies to help adults become engaged and perhaps even enjoy the learning activities. First, consider how the information is presented. Instead of showing the same video to the same participants year after year, develop some creative teaching strategies. Perhaps a game, group discussion, crossword puzzle, or simulation can accomplish the same goal.

Next, analyze the content. Can you provide new and interesting facts? Work to establish a need to know. Adults learn best when they feel that the information is relevant and applicable. For example, begin a fire safety discussion by sharing news clips of fires in other health care facilities, and begin a group discussion about how a similar fire could be handled at your facility.

8. How can I motivate nurses to want to learn?

Essentially five characteristics and skills have been shown to motivate learning:

1. **Expertise, knowledge, and preparation.** Learners need to recognize that the instructor knows something that is beneficial and useful to them. Nurses come with experiences that may surpass those of the instructor. Ask nurses to share experiences related to the content. Encouraging their active participation in discussion conveys your appreciation of their experience—a real motivator! You also must provide nurses with concrete examples that they can understand, use, and apply. Explain or demonstrate why they would want to learn the information. Provide information that is not readily available to them in other ways. One error frequently made by instructors is to reteach what is in the book. This approach erodes the instructor's credibility and destroys the mutual respect that is essential for a healthy learner-teacher relationship. Next, know the content and subject well. Knowledge enhances your confidence, flexibility, and creativity. No longer is the instructor relegated to lecture; group discussion, games, and other innovative teaching strategies are a possibility. Finally, be prepared. Not only should you know the content well, but also it is a good idea to have back-up plans to address different learning styles.

2. **Empathy.** One of the keys to motivating adults is the need for empathy. Adults come with a variety of experiences, concerns, and needs. They come to learning activities for specific reasons. Adults' needs and expectations for what they are taught powerfully influence how they respond to what they are taught. Adapt your instruction to the learners' level of experience and skill development. Give participants activities that are within their reach, but not so easily mastered that they become bored. Continuously consider the learners' perspective, and respond to their concerns.

3. **Attitude.** One of the best motivators is the teacher's enthusiasm for the course, the students, and the subject matter. Enthusiastic presenters are more believable, and nurses will want to listen. Instructors must care about and value what they teach for themselves as well as for the learners. The commitment to the group must be evident. It is expressed in the instruction by using appropriate degrees of emotion, animation, and energy. Practice using these eight indicators of high teacher enthusiasm[8]:

- Rapid, uplifting, varied vocal delivery
- Dancing, wide open eyes
- Frequent, demonstrative gestures
- Varied, dramatic body movements
- Varied, emotive facial expressions

- Selection of varied words, especially adjectives
- Ready, animated acceptance of ideas and feelings
- Exuberant energy level

4. **Effectiveness.** People seldom learn what they cannot understand. Instructional clarity means teaching something in a manner that is easy for learners to comprehend and that is organized so that they can smoothly follow the intended lesson or program. Use words that the learners understand, and avoid vagueness. Describe precisely, and give appropriate examples. Be organized in the presentation. The discussion should be a road map, with a preplanned destination. This is not to say that you cannot use an alternate route—flexibility is important, but this, too, must be preplanned. Provide ways for learners to comprehend what has been said if it was not clear in the initial presentation. Most importantly, remember that effective teaching is a learned behavior. Continuously strive to improve the effectiveness of your presentation.[8]

5. **Reinforcement.** Reinforcement improves retention of information. Positive reinforcement increases participation throughout an event. Removal of negative and threatening consequences also motivates learners. For example, if a nurse who asks a question in a class is humiliated by giggles from peers, she is not likely to ask questions in the future. Instead, responding with enthusiasm, acceptance, and praise is likely to promote the nurse's willingness to ask additional questions and contribute to the discussion.

9. How should an educator deal with rude, disruptive, and uncooperative students?

As instructors of adults, we generally expect that nurses will be well behaved and attentive. Unfortunately, at times we may encounter a participant who is uncooperative or disruptive, for whatever reason. The best way to handle the situation is to be respectful, yet directive and assertive. It is generally most helpful to speak to the person individually during a break so as not to demean him or her. While waiting for a break, you may find it effective to call on the disruptive person to answer a question or to participate in the group discussion. "Roaming" around the classroom is also helpful, because participants tend to be more attentive if you are standing near them. Most importantly, be sure to outline the expectations at the onset of the program, and be sure to assess learning needs. Nurses come to an educational session with expectations for the program. Find out what those expectations are, and then enthusiastically present the content that meets their learning needs. A good strategy is to begin the session by asking participants what their expectations for the class are.

10. What is a self-directed learning activity?

In a self-directed learning activity, the learner takes initiative and responsibility for the learning process. Examples of self-directed learning activities include informal investigation, self-guided focused readings, computer-assisted learning, distance learning, directed readings, and programmed instruction. Self-directed activities do not eliminate the need for the staff development educator. Instead, the educator assumes the role of facilitator, assisting learners to explore and discover answers to their questions. Programmed texts are available for courses such as medical terminology and EKG rhythm recognition. Staff can take these courses at their own pace; however it is helpful for an instructor to provide support and feedback as well as answer questions.

11. How is my role as an educator different if I use adult learning principles?

Educators using adult learning principles assume different roles from those in the traditional teaching environment. Adult learners are provided with considerably more freedom and responsibility for course planning, implementation, and evaluation. Use of adult learning principles actively involves participants and stimulates use of a broader variety of resources as learners work collaboratively with others to achieve their personal learning goals. Because adults are self-directed, they tend to be more accountable for their actions in this type of setting. Consequently, the instructor is more of a facilitator than a content expert who lectures about his or her knowledge to passive students. Nurses are expected to be active participants in the learning process.

The staff development educator, working collaboratively with the staff, develops learning activities that are as close as possible to actual practice; the applicability to practice becomes obvious.

Learning activities are a reflection of past and current experiences so that nurses can use and build upon valuable experiences. Sequence the course material according to staff's readiness to learn. Learning activities may be individualized and include various techniques, such as lab experiences, simulations, and independent study. Finally, evaluation is largely a reflective practice. Learners evaluate how they are progressing toward their goals and how they might better accomplish the course objectives. Adult education requires use of a collaborative and democratic style of teaching.

12. Is there any truth to the adage, "You can't teach an old dog new tricks"?

Perhaps the most important aspect of adult learning theory is the instructor's understanding of adult learners. Physiologically, psychologically, cognitively, and sociologically, adults are a diverse group. Many people incorrectly believe that older adults have little, if any, ability to learn. Older adults can and do learn skills and information and are able to apply immediately what they have learned.

Intelligence testing indicates that the ability to solve new problems declines with age, but crystallized intelligence, which is based on learning and experience, may increase or is at least maintained. However, the key to teaching older adults, as with all populations, is careful assessment of learning needs, style, and ability.

13. What steps can I take to build an educational environment conducive to adult learners?

The intrinsic differences of adults, which can be attributed to previous learning experiences, abilities, and motivation, are important components for the instructor to address at the onset of a program. For example, a participant who has had previous difficulty in passing a certification course may come to a review session with a high level of anxiety. In addition, adults have many situations in their lives competing for their attention (such as work, family, and life circumstances). Knowles[6] states that the educational environment established by the instructor should include learning that is problem-centered and experience-centered. It is crucial to create an environment that is relaxed and psychologically safe while developing a climate of trust and mutual respect.

Creating an Environment Conducive to Adult Learning

PRINCIPLE OF EFFECTIVE PRACTICE	IMPLICATIONS FOR PRACTICE
Voluntary participation. Adults' motivation to learn is naturally high; because participants engage voluntarily in activities, their active participation can be withdrawn quickly and easily if they feel that the activity does not meet their needs.	Expend a high level of effort and ingenuity in preparing for each class. Adults are less likely to resist teaching techniques that are participatory and experiential, such as discussion, role-play, games, and small group work, if they understand and have had regular exposure to creative teaching techniques.
Mutual respect. Adult learners need to be valued as unique individuals deserving respect.	Ensure that the climate and culture of learning is safe. Recognize participants for past experiences and accomplishments regularly. Establish rules and expectations at the start of the program, and follow through with enforcement of the rules. Keep the pace of the content fast enough to meet the time expectations of learners and to keep them interested, but slow enough to cover the information and ensure understanding. Handle disruptive situations. Provide a comfortable environment. Establish an environment in which negotiation of expectations is encouraged. Allow participants to progress at their own pace. Be available privately to assist participants having difficulty with the content.

Continued on following page

Creating an Environment Conducive to Adult Learning (Continued)

PRINCIPLE OF EFFECTIVE PRACTICE	IMPLICATIONS FOR PRACTICE
Action/reflection. Adults need time to learn and then reflect on their learning before new learning occurs.	Apply new ideas, skills, and concepts in the context of past, current, and future learning as much as possible.
Self-direction. Adults strive to be self-directed problem solvers. The role of educator is not only to teach the content but also to promote a movement toward independent learning.	Progressively strive to decrease dependence on the instructor while maintaining a safe environment. Help learners understand and use available resources. Assist learners to identify their own learning needs. Allow nurses to assume increasing responsibility for planning programs. Foster decision-making by teaching problem-solving and critical analysis. Provide frequent reinforcement. Emphasize experiential, participatory, proactive instructional methods.

14. Adult learning theory promotes active and participatory teaching methods. Can instructors still use lecture as a teaching method?

Absolutely. Adult learning theory signifies a change in the understanding of adult learners and approach to the education of adults. All teaching methods, including lecture, can be effectively used to teach adults. The key is that the learning activity is more self-directed and less teacher-directed. Adults learn more deeply and retain better when they learn what they want, when they want, on their own initiative. The difference between pedagogic and andragogic education is not so much the difference in the underlying theory as the difference in the attitude of the learners. If self-directed learners recognize that on occasion they will be "taught to," using methods such as lecture, they will enter the situation in a searching, probing frame of mind. The learners will begin to view traditional "passive" learning experiences as resources for enrichment without losing their self-directedness.

15. In what situations is it acceptable for a learner to assume a dependent role?

The learner must assume a dependent role when the content is entirely new. In such situations, past experiences may be of little worth. The instructor can promote active learning by asking stimulating or controversial questions, promoting group discussions, or demonstrating the procedure. The key for both instructor and students is that the self-directed learner participates in development of and controls the learning variables.

16. List some of the important learning variables.

- Identification of learning needs
- Topic or activity
- Expected outcomes
- Approaches and alternative learning experiences
- Learning resources
- Time, pace, and environment
- Method of evaluation
- Method of documentation

17. As a staff development educator, I am often frustrated by the lack of involvement of participants in the educational process. Can you offer suggestions?

Indeed, young adults of the present are different from those of the past. They have been programmed through many years of formal education to be passive, dependent learners. Parents, teachers, and even school systems have accepted responsibility for student learning rather than requiring learners to be accountable for acquiring the needed information. Society is also quite different. Adults value free time and have instantaneous access to a wealth of information at their fingertips. Therefore, the information presented must be succinct and applicable to capture and maintain their interest. Educators who are unfamiliar with the characteristics of adult learners see contemporary students as underprepared or less intelligent and motivated than previous generations. The result is a sense of disappointment and frustration in both learners and teachers.

These frustrations have resulted in a strong push toward the increased use of andragogic principles—a push to make students desire to be lifelong learners, to be active learners, and to be partners in the educational process. We must remember, however, that the learner is responsible for his or her own learning. As educators, we provide the tools, opportunities, and resources for success. We can assist people to become active learners by providing a variety of learning activities such as role-playing, simulations, group discussions, and independent learning projects. However, the decision to use the opportunities is in the hand of the learner.

18. Can an educator whose employer does not use andragogic principles effectively integrate adult learning theory in his or her teaching?

If only everyone subscribed to adult teaching principles—but many have not. Even if an educator is employed in a setting that promotes and encourages pedagogic behavior, he or she possesses the ability to promote lifelong learning in others. This goal can be accomplished by using and promoting active, participatory roles in the classroom, by collaborating with students, by demonstrating and using reflective thinking, and by empowering learners whenever possible. Most importantly, proponents of adult learning theory can encourage dialogue about the usefulness of the educational process. Even nonbelievers will recognize that acceptance, respect, and empathy are positive characteristics for an educator. Most administrators will be supportive of many adult learning principles, and many adult learners will be appreciative of the learning process. Remind your administrators tactfully that there is more than one way to teach well and that a theory does not have to be universally accepted to be useful in practice.[4]

19. Some students seem to be more comfortable with lectures instead of the more creative styles of presentation. Is this a normal characteristic of adult learners?

Adult learners tend to expect learning to be delivered in the traditional, teacher-led method to which they have been exposed over the years. To preserve self-esteem, adult learners want a safe, nonthreatening environment. A lecture format provides safety but may not be the most effective teaching method. Introduce new teaching formats gradually. A combination of lecture and discussion, especially when the instructor uses Power Point or other presentation software, can be highly effective. If the participants seem to prefer a lecture format, incorporate a Socratic approach (asking application and analysis-level questions) to stimulate discussion and engage learners. Sharing your clinical experiences also livens the approach and helps learners to make important connections.

20. I teach adults of various abilities and educational levels simultaneously. Should I teach at a more basic level in a particular group to ensure that all participants understand?

This challenge is commonly encountered by educators. In every course, the staff development educator faces students of different competencies, experiences, and abilities. If the instructor chooses to teach to the rudimentary student, the more advanced students will not be challenged. On the other hand, the instructor who chooses to teach at a higher level sufficient to challenge advanced students risks losing students who are having difficulty. This dilemma speaks directly to the usefulness and need to use adult learning theory in continuing education settings. As many have discovered, not all adults are alike. This question is a classic representation of problems inherent to teacher-controlled settings.

To resolve the issue, first acknowledge the experience of everyone in the group. Second, encourage students to develop personal learning contracts that identify what they wish to acquire from the course and how they will achieve their goals. Next, try to develop learning activities and teaching methods that provide an avenue for all students to excel. This approach may include small group work, independent assignments, or self-study instructional packets. By using these techniques, the instructor permits each student to work at his or her own pace. Students who can move through the information quickly do so until they reach a topic that is more challenging. Students who encounter difficulty are permitted to move more slowly and can seek help from available resources, including the instructor and others in the class. This approach also allows the facilitator to provide individual feedback in a positive manner. Participants who have developed personal learning contracts can complete self-assessments to determine progress toward their goals. The important point is to accomplish the objectives identified at the onset of the program—not the process of how students reach their goals.

21. I understand adult learning theory and andragogic principles but have difficulty in applying them to continuing education. How can I use them in my practice?

A case study may help. I had been assigned to teach a cardiac dysrhythmia interpretation course to a group of people with varied experiences. The class included lay people with no cardiac rhythm knowledge or experience, caregivers with various licensure and certification levels (e.g., RNs, LPNs, respiratory therapists) with little or no cardiac experience, and cardiac care providers with extensive experience. Attendance at the course was mandatory for all students. The table below contains a sample plan and framework used to accomplish the course goals. The plan was developed at the onset of the training program, with the recognition that the course would be met with resistance by some and fear by others. Following this framework, additional unit lesson plans were developed.

Sample Motivational Plan Using Andragogic Principles

Instructional objective: At the end of the program, learners will be able to identify cardiac rhythm disturbances with 100% accuracy.

PRINCIPLE	DISCUSSION	LEARNING ACTIVITY/INSTRUCTIONAL BEHAVIOR
Self-direction	As adults mature, they move to self-directing behavior. They are responsible for their own learning.	1. At the onset of the program, students complete an *individualized instruction plan.* The instructor helps each student to develop his or her plan, which includes the following: • Identification of personal learning needs • Selection of specific focus for the project (i.e., a statement of purpose related to professional competence) • Determination of expected, measurable outcomes • Identification of possible learning resources • Determination of evaluation methods 2. The facilitator helps students to identify organizational and individual competency needs. 3. The facilitator creates a learning environment in which those competencies and goals can be attained. 4. The facilitator provides employees with an understanding of why it is to their benefit to take advantage of the resources offered. The facilitator establishes a need to know.
Experience	All adults come with valuable and useful experiences. The goal is positive recognition of the value and experience of all participants.	1. Acknowledge and share that the participants themselves are the richest resource for one another. • Use teaching strategies that promote group experiences, such as group discussions, simulations, games, and problem-solving projects. 2. Differences in experiences ensure heterogeneity in the group. Using individualized learning contracts, develop assignments and projects for each student: • What do you want to learn from this class? • How will you know when you have learned it?
Readiness to learn	Adults become ready to learn when they experience a need to know. The goal is to help students identify what and why they need to know.	1. Assist experienced participants to identify gaps in knowledge using a variety of techniques, such as preassessment tests and questionnaires, to assist in developing personal goals. 2. Assist all providers in identifying the process for addressing the gaps in knowledge.

Continued on following page

Sample Motivational Plan Using Andragogic Principles (Cont.)

PRINCIPLE	DISCUSSION	LEARNING ACTIVITY/INSTRUCTIONAL BEHAVIOR
Orientation to learning	Learning experiences should be organized around life situations rather than subject units. The goal is to establish clear expectations and guidelines for the learning process.	1. Establish group learning goals collaboratively, but be willing to negotiate as needed. 2. Recognize the need to acknowledge life roles that compete with the educational process. 3. Make the learning activity immediately applicable and relevant. Include realistic situations in case scenarios and clinical rotations, and encourage participation by everyone in all activities. 4. Develop both group and independent learning activities to permit participants to progress at their own pace.
Motivation	Adults are naturally motivated to learn. The goal is to maintain and develop motivation throughout the program by addressing attitude, learning needs, stimulation and interest, and feedback.	1. Demonstrate enthusiasm. 2. Confront false beliefs about potential course difficulties. 3. Establish course rules. 4. Create an environment conducive to learning: • Safe, nonthreatening • Comfortable • Address psychosocial and physical needs of each participant. 5. Organize a tutorial assistance plan for all participants—a safety net for those having difficulty. 6. Help students to identify and accomplish their learning needs. 7. Establish expectations and rules at the onset. 8. Reinforce need for personal learning plans so that each can progress at his or her own pace. 9. Vary teaching strategies; use games, create problem-solving activities, and present real-life situations to challenge students of all levels. 10. Organize teaching systematically (i.e., simple to complex). 11. Encourage and promote active participation. 12. Alternate roles in group work. 13. Provide feedback regularly, using a variety of methods: verbal public praise, written comments, recognition for accomplishments. 14. Offer constructive criticism discreetly. 15. Build self-confidence by recognizing successful completion of progressive objectives. 16. Continually reinforce improvement in quality of life and life roles.

BIBLIOGRAPHY

1. Bastable SS: Nurse as Educator: Principles of Teaching and Learning. Sudbury, MA, Jones & Bartlett, 1997.
2. Brookfield SD: Understanding and Facilitating Adult Learning, San Francisco, Jossey-Bass, 1986.
3. Campbell KN: Adult education: Helping adults begin the process of learning. AAHON J 47:31–42, 1999.
4. Grow GO: Teaching learners to be self-directed. Adult Educ Q 41:3, 125–149, 1991.
5. Knowles MS: Andragogy in Action. San Francisco, Jossey Bass, 1984.
6. Knowles MS: The Modern Practice of Adult Education: From Pedagogy to Andragogy, Englewood Cliffs, NJ, Prentice Hall Regents, 1980, pp 40–45.
7. Milligan F: In defense of andragogy. Nurse Educ Today 15:22–27, 1995.
8. Wlodkowski RJ: Strategies to enhance adult motivation to learn. In Galbraith MW (ed): Adult Learning Methods: A Guide for Effective Instruction. Malabar, FL, Krieger Publishing, 1990, pp 97–188.

13. DEALING WITH DIVERSITY IN LEARNERS

Cheryl B. *Robinson*, RN, BSN, MSN, *and Kristen* L. O'*Shea*, MS, RN

1. In what ways is diversity an issue in the education setting?

As an educator, you need to be aware of all of the possible ways in which the diversity of learners affects the way they learn. Leininger states that ethnicity, religion, education, age, gender, and acculturation can influence the educational setting.[10] In addition, great differences exist in the ways that people learn, think, and react to change. An awareness of these differences can help you to create an optimal learning environment for all learners.

2. What are the different learning styles?

Several theories or models attempt to explain the ways in which people learn new knowledge and skills. Kolb designed a framework for determining individual strengths and weaknesses in learning. Kolb's model lists the types of learners as convergers, divergers, assimilators, and accommodaters.[8] The following chart summarizes Kolb's work and incorporates learning strategies and evaluation methods.

	CONVERGER	DIVERGER	ASSIMILATOR	ACCOMMODATOR
Learning modes	Kinesthetic; Thinking	Visual; Feeling	Visual; Thinking	Kinesthetic; Feeling
Strengths	Standardized tests; finding practical uses for theories and ideas	Views situations from different viewpoints; interpersonally oriented	Understands masses of information; logical thinking; creation of theoretical models	Flexible; takes risks; learns by doing; likes challenges
Best learning strategies	Memorization; programmed instruction; return demonstrations; mastery learning	Personal and social awareness; small group work; communications	Independent study; concept formation; problem-solving; comprehensive planning	Case studies; skills lab; self-expression; values clarification; imagination
Individual characteristics	Realistic, practical, matter of fact	Friendly, sympathetic	Intellectual, logical	Imaginative, insightful, curious
Evaluation procedures	Demonstration of skills; objective tests	Self-reporting, personal journals	Essays, demonstration of ability to analyze	Elaboration to detail; producing creative products
Environmental	Organization; purposeful work	Interaction; collaboration	Discovery and independence	Originality, flexibility

Hermann proposes that we have four primary quadrants of the brain. He has created a model that uses research about the right and left brain to demonstrate how each person uses his or her brain in the process of thinking and learning. He divides the brain into quadrants as follows:

Upper left (cerebral): rational self — **Upper right** (cerebral): experimental self

Lower left (limbic): safe-keeping self — **Lower right** (limbic): feeling self

Each person is believed to have a dominant quadrant of the brain. According to Hermann, the brain is the source of who we are and how we learn. For example, Hermann believes that right-dominant people are emotional and learn best by kinesthetic means. In nurses and people-oriented individuals, the dominant quadrant is most likely the lower right. Hermann believes that most health services educators have a lower left-dominant "safe-keeping self" style and are highly detailed and organized.[7] The differences between the right- and left-dominant styles may lead to conflict in learning and understanding from the educator.

Finally, Gregorc developed a concept of learning styles that is based on dualities of ordering (sequentially or randomly) and perceiving information (abstractly or concretely).[5] He also identified four styles of learning preferences: concrete sequential, abstract sequential, abstract random, and concrete random. Each of these styles has certain characteristics. When a concrete sequential learner is paired with an abstract random learner, conflict results.

3. Why do I need to assess learning styles?

An educator, who understands the dynamics of the learning styles,can implement strategies to encourage individual learning and at the same time balance the learning needs of the entire group. You should be able to present an educational program that uses diverse methods. Diversity in presentation, including audio, video, visual aids, activities, and role playing, provides multiple channels for learning.

Probably the greatest diversity issue that educators encounter is the diversity in thinking and learning styles. You must understand the learner's needs and struggles with n the educational setting. The following chart, describing Hermann's thinking styles, attempts to place these expectations, struggles, and characteristics into context:

	RATIONAL SELF	EXPERIMENTAL SELF	SAFE-KEEPING SELF	FEELING SELF
Expectations	Precise information, theory rationales, textbook readings, proof of validity	Fun and spontaneity, discovery of content, quick pace, new ideas and concepts	Organized approach, staying on track, examples, clear instructions	Group discussions; express feelings, hands-on learning, kinesthetic
Challenges in learning	Lack of logic, imprecise with concepts and ideas, expressing emotion	Time management, administration and detail, lack of flexibility	Risk taking, ambiguity, unclear directions	Too much data, pure lecture, lack of participation
Characteristics	Knows how things are, likes numbers, realistic and logical, analyzes and quantifies	Imagines, curious, breaks rules, speculates, takes risks	Plans, timely, neat, organizes, reliable, establishes procedures, gets things done	Expressive, supportive, talks a lot, emotional, feels, likes to teach, sensitive to others

By learning about the diversity of the participants in an educational setting, you can develop activities, programs, and settings that reach all learning styles and enable the learners to gain the most from the learning experience and from their study or practice time. Although you should be aware of learning styles, labeling can have its drawbacks. Labeling involves the danger of missing some of the multiple preferences in the group or in focusing on a single style or teaching method.

4. How can I assess learning style?

First, you should gain understanding of the characteristics of the different learning styles. In face-to-face delivery, the learning culture can be assessed quickly. The educator can identify the characteristics of the employees that combine to create the group dynamics. Getting to know the participants is the initial step in creating learning culture. As many have said, "First impressions are often lasting impressions." The main point is that the program can be planned by the educator, but the employee/student controls the flow of the information. Therefore, the employees or students begin to establish the tone of the learning experience early in the process and mold the course of the learning experience.

Adult learners have unique patterns. Look for the participants who tend to be practical and structured in approach. They are most likely concrete thinkers, and their learning experiences need to focus on content. Participants who tend to be analytical and evaluative prefer to work alone; cooperative activities are stressful for them. They are abstract and need validation from the leader and direction to pertinent resources. By understanding these different styles of learning, the educator can mold an atmosphere of learning for all types of learners.

5. What guides are available to examine the principles of adult learning styles?

Conti created the Principle of Adult Learning Scale (PALS),[4] which is designed to find better ways to help adults learn and to help educators and staff developers more effectively guide the educational experience. When using this or any other guide, remember that you are dealing with a multitude of learning styles. There may be as many as twenty-five different learning tools that can guide the developer to educational programs conducive to meeting the needs of adult learners.

6. How does learning style affect learning in the educational setting?

Educators must remember that all learners retain knowledge in differing ways. Active learners tend to retain knowledge best through "hands-on" experience or explaining it to others. Intuitive learners like to discover relationships and hate repetition. Visual learners prefer diagrams and charts, and sequential learners tend to follow logical paths. Lastly, global learners are people who learn in large amounts but have difficulty explaining how they learned what they learned. All of these types of these learners may be lumped into the educational setting at one time.

7. How can I motivate a diverse group of learners?

Adults are motivated by what has personal meaning for them. Most are motivated by the pragmatic desire to use or apply some newly available knowledge or skill. You must perform an assessment to prioritize the needs and interests of the learners (see Chapter 8). The information gained by the assessment can be used to guide you in setting objectives and planning teaching strategies. Learning styles of the participants and the potential dynamics of a group of diverse learners need to be considered in the planning stage.

Wlodkowski describes six factors that can affect motivation[13]: attitude, need, stimulation, affect, competencies, and reinforcement. Reinforcement continues the learning process, and you are the reinforcer. Reinforcement may be different for different types of learners. As the reinforcer, you must provide guidance, which is seen by the learner as motivating professional maturity and mastery.

8. List some simple steps to appeal to different learning styles in an educational setting.

- Assess the abilities of the students.
- Provide individualized instruction.
- Provide a safe environment, so that mistakes are part of the learning process.
- Allow small group discussion to encourage feedback.
- Provide independent learning experiences.
- Incorporate different approaches, such as lecture, audiovisual aids, and examples.
- Provide opportunities for demonstration to appeal to visual learners.
- Involve students to allow them to feel part of the course—lead discussions.
- Introduce role-playing to help incorporate cognitive learning and evaluation.

In teaching, the challenge is to make a meaningful connection with each individual learner. Unfortunately, there is no magic formula. Some learners profit from a visual approach, others from physical activities, and still others from a verbal approach. But most learn from a combination of approaches.

9. What is a learning disability?

A learning disability is a neurologic disorder that causes difficulties in learning. The Learning Disabilities Association offers the following definition:

> a chronic condition of presumed neurological origin which selectively interferes with the development, integration and/or demonstration of verbal and nonverbal abilities. Specific learning disabilities exist as a distinct handicapping condition in the presence of average to superior intelligence, adequate sensory and motor systems, and adequate learning opportunities. The condition varies in its manifestations and in the degree of severity throughout life. The condition can affect self-esteem, education, vocation, socialization, and daily living activities.

These disorders must not be associated with low intelligence, poor motivation, or inadequate teaching. Learning disabilities may be seen in language (either spoken or written form) and in arithmetic. Approximately 10% of the American population experiences some type of learning disability.[12]

10. How can I assess for a learning disability?

Employees in your class may come to you voluntarily to report a previously diagnosed learning disability. Try to gain as much information as possible. Ask if they have any material that may assist you in helping them. Although many adults may experience difficulties in learning from time to time, a consistent pattern of behaviors over time can clue an educator that a problem may exist. The following characteristics or behaviors may indicate a learning difficulty:

- Trouble with remembering newly learned information
- Problems with understanding what is read
- Inability to stay organized
- Difficulty expressing thoughts orally or in writing
- Problems with remembering or sticking to deadlines
- Difficulty following directions
- Inappropriate remarks
- Trouble with getting along with peers or coworkers

11. What specific strategies can I use to deal with staff who have disabilities?

Educators must follow a manageable list of activities to help staff with learning disabilities to be more comfortable in the educational setting. The following are specific suggestions:

- Encourage peer tutoring and cooperative learning.
- Help learners get organized.
- Give learners with disabilities extra time for testing or skills.
- Allow tape recorders so that notes can be more complete.
- Do not put learners with disabilities under the stress of time or competition.
- Be aware of your own communication styles.
- Follow as structured a schedule as possible.
- Convey a positive attitude about learners with disabilities.
- Provide clear and concise written instructions.
- Praise always encourages others.

12. What if the learning disability is so great that job performance is affected?

Under the Americans with Disabilities Act (ADA), as an employer you must make reasonable accommodations. If you have difficulty in finding learning support and teaching methods to help employees with disabilities learn their job, seek the help of the human resources department. A full evaluation may be needed to determine the exact nature of the learning disability and its effect on the employee. The employee assistance program (EAP) or behavioral services department can make recommendations for a psychologist's evaluation. All reasonable efforts need to be made to assist the employee who is a student in your class.

13. I have a nursing assistant with partial loss of hearing. What should I do?

It is certainly possible for the nursing assistant with partial loss of hearing to perform his or her job. You must determine what assistance is necessary to help the nurse succeed in your class. You need to evaluate the thoroughness of your written hand-outs. Be sure that you use plenty of visual aids to support what you are saying. It is possible to purchase an amplified stethoscope for listening to blood pressures. (Under the ADA this would be considered a reasonable accommodation.)

14. What effect does age have on learning?

It was once thought that learning is for the younger generations and that "old dogs can't learn new tricks." The evidence over the years, however, shows that the aging process need not be considered a major handicap in learning. Although aging encompasses a wide variety of physical changes, reaction time, vision, and hearing are the three changes most likely to interfere with learning. Speed of learning involves reaction time to perceive the stimulus, transmission time, and response time to carry out the action. A generalized slowing down accompanies aging, but educators need to ask a fundamental question: At what age does slowing down of cognitive function have any practical effect on learning ability? Speed is the basic concept involved. One interesting finding concludes that there is a rise in intelligence to the mid 40s and a high plateau into the mid 50s.[13]

Youth are geared toward acquisition of skills, young adults are major achievers, middle-aged adults tend to take on major life responsibilities, and older adults look at reintegration of thoughts and skills. You should keep these developmental stages in mind when you are dealing with a class of learners from a variety of age groups.

15. Does generation affect the way in which students learn?

Absolutely. You may want to read *Generations at Work: Managing the Clash of Veterans, Boomers, Xers and Nexters in Your Workplace* by Zemke, Raines, and Filipczak. The book is a guide to practical solutions to managing the age-diverse workplace. The following chart summarizes the four generational groups and their learning characteristics.

GENERATION	YEARS OF BIRTH	LEARNING IMPLICATIONS
Veterans	1922–1943	Respond well to traditional classroom with lectures and presentations by topic experts. Like information that is organized, well researched, and supported by facts and figures. Dislike situations in which they may be made to look foolish. Training material should be in a large font with a simple format. On-the-job training works well if it is respectful, nonthreatening, and risk-free.
Boomers	1943–1960	Value lifelong learning and view education as a means to climb the ladder. Like team-building sessions. Like self-learning (videos, audio tapes, self-learning packets). Like materials that include plenty of information (resources for later).
Xers	1960–1980	Value education highly. More comfortable than others with computers. Like CD-ROM, interactive video, distance learning, and Internet courses. Like a highly interactive classroom with role-playing and coaching. Like busy attention-getting hand-outs.
Nexters or Millennials	1980–2000	Are just joining the the workforce. Read more than Xers. Used to learning in highly interactive ways.

16. Some recently hired nursing assistant students come from challenging home situations and often lack previous work experience. How can I help them acclimate to the work force?

You have a golden opportunity to make a difference in the lives of the staff that you teach. Entry level staff often lack the background experience and education to prepare them for the health care setting. You may take for granted that all staff have basic social and work skills, but this may not be the case for entry-level employees. You may assume, for example, that everyone knows how to set an alarm clock and how to get to work on time. Many people, however, have not been taught these simple skills, and incorporating some of them into your training may be necessary.

It is important to treat each of your students with respect. You may be surprised to find out what kinds of home situations your students are coming from. Setting clear classroom expectations is necessary and assists your students in preparing for the work setting. Remember that this may be their first formal classroom experience since high school. It may be necessary to assist with study skills. It also may be necessary to teach problem-solving skills for dealing with work-home balance and to give suggestions about how to deal with childcare and other daily issues.

17. Usually I enjoy my role as an educator. Once in a while, however, a participant in my class is difficult to deal with. What should I do?

Several types of participants can be difficult to deal with in the classroom setting. However, according to Pike, you should keep in mind two essential actions when dealing with any type of difficult participant: (1) get the participant on board, and (2) minimize his or her effect on the group. The following table outlines some of the specific steps you can take to deal with difficult behaviors in your classroom.

PARTICIPANT BEHAVIOR	STRATEGIES FOR DEALING WITH DIFFICULT BEHAVIOR
Know-it-all who challenges your credibility	Ask to hear other participants' feedback and answers. Confront the issue in private. Ignore the behavior. Try to maintain your composure.
One or two participants who do all of the talking	Show respect for their contributions. Interrupt (with tact) and redirect discussion to others in group. Make eye contact with another participant and move discussion to that person. Call a break to change the flow of the class. Discuss the situation in private with the participants and enlist their help (ask them to wait for others to speak first or count to ten before speaking). Ask to hear other participants' thoughts. ("Let's see what everyone else has to say about this." You may need to switch to a more lecture-type format. Offer tokens for participation. When the tokens are gone, the participant is finished participating. Consider assigning jobs within the group, or assign people to answer questions. Rotate the leadership of the group.
Quiet person who does not participate	Discuss in private to identify issues that affect participation. Ask the participant a specific question. Make direct eye contact. Give positive reinforcement for contributions. Appoint the person to be group leader.
Participant who does not want to be there	Be sure to make your case for why the person is there and "what's in it for me." Identify the issue up font, and enlist the person's assistance in making the class a worthwhile experience.

Continued on following page

PARTICIPANT BEHAVIOR	STRATEGIES FOR DEALING WITH DIFFICULT BEHAVIOR
Chatty participants who have a side conversation	Look at them. Ask the group if all can hear the speaker. Walk over and stand near them. Ask a question of a participant who is nearby so that the discussion is in close proximity to the talkers. As a last resort, stop and wait for quiet.

BIBLIOGRAPHY

1. Americans with Disabilities Act: What is a learning disability? Available at http://www.usdoj.gov/crt/ada/learnfac.htm.
2. Bastable SB: Nurse As Educator. Boston, Jones & Bartlett, 1997.
3. Botwinick J: Intellectual abilities. In Birren JE, Schaie KW (eds): Handbook of the Psychology of Aging. New York, Van Nostrand-Reinhold, 1977.
4. Conti GJ: Identifying your teaching style. In MW Galbraith (ed): Adult Learning Methods for Effective Instructions. Malabar, FL, Krieger, 1990, pp 79–96.
5. Gregorc AF: An Adult's Guide to Style. Maynard, MA, Gabriel Systems,1982, p 40.
6. Hegyvary ST: From diversity to enrichment. J Prof Nurs 8:261, 1992.
7. Hermann N: The Creative Brain. Lake Lure, NC, Brain Books, 1988.
8. Kolb DA: LSI-IIa: Self Scoring Inventory and Interpretation Booklet. Boston, McBer, 1993.
9. Krathwohl DR, et al: Taxonomy of Education Objectives, the Classification of Educational Goals. Handbook 2: The Affective Domain. New York, Longman, 1964.
10. Leininger MM: Transcultural Nursing: Concepts, Theory, Research, and Practice, 2nd ed. Columbus, OH, McGraw-Hill & Greyden Press, 1995.
11. Pike RW: Dealing with difficult participants. Available at http://www.creativetrainingtech. com/support/free/deep/dealing.html
12. Soloman BA, Felder RM: Learning styles and strategies. Available at http://cte.uncwil.edu/soloman_felder.htm
13. Trough AM: The other 80 percent of learning. In Gross R (Ed): An Invitation to Lifelong Learning. Atlanta, Follett, 1971, pp 20–22.
14. Wlodkowski RJ: Enhancing Adult Motivation to Learn. San Francisco, Jossey-Bass, 1985.
15. Zemke R et al: Generations at Work. New York, AMACOM, 2000.

14. PRESENTATION SKILLS

Barbara L. Paterson, PhD, RN

1. What tips do you have for an inexperienced presenter?

- Organize your presentation beforehand. Few audiences will recognize the value of what you have to say if your presentation is scattered and disorganized.
- Your lecture is going to be heard, not read. Use a conversational tone with short, straightforward sentences and simple words whenever you can.
- Try to maintain an even pace throughout the presentation. If you go too fast or too slow, you will lose the audience's attention.
- Lecture for no longer than 10–20 minutes at a time (the average attention span of adults). After 15 minutes or so, change the teaching strategy (e.g., show a film clip or ask audience members to share their stories about the topic).
- Never present from a verbatim script. Presenters who rely greatly on their notes or those who memorize their presentation often lose their place and appear unnatural and uninviting in their presentations.
- If you have to read something, make sure that it is no longer than 10 lines in length. Put it on an overhead projection or slide so that the audience can read it along with you.
- Plan the questions that you will ask during and after the presentation. If you phrase questions in a vague or unclear way, you can often frustrate and annoy the audience.
- Rehearse with someone who can be trusted to give you credible feedback and suggestions about your presentation style. Ask the person to watch for mannerisms and patterns of speech that may detract from the effectiveness of the presentation, such as dropping the voice tone at the end of sentences, finger tapping, or frequent "ums" between sentences. It helps if you record yourself speaking, noting how many times you practice these habits. Then develop a way of attending to such habits while you speak (I always listen to myself as I am speaking) and pausing before you feel yourself about to say a "hmmm" or do something that will distract the listeners, such as tapping your fingers. Do not overrehearse, however; your presentation may sound stale.
- If you make mistakes or do not know the answer to a question, admit it gracefully and with humor. Most audiences will be supportive.

2. What should I do if I have little interest or enthusiasm for the topic?

When a presenter seems uninterested in the topic, the audience tends to be bored. In most cases, it is best to teach what you know and love. However, sometimes you may be asked to speak about something in which you have little interest. On such occasions you need to find ways of making the topic interesting to you. You need to stir up some passion for the subject. I was asked to deliver a presentation about enemas to nursing students. It was definitely not my topic of interest. In preparation for the presentation, I interviewed nurses who had graduated from 1920 to 1930 about their experiences with enemas. The stories were often hilarious and sometimes tragic. The nurses told many stories about people's creative use of household materials for enema tubing and recipes for nurses to cook up a batch of enema solution. These stories formed the basis of the presentation and helped me to feel a passion for the subject that I did not feel beforehand.

3. How should I organize the presentation?

There are a number of ways of organizing the content of a presentation. For example, you may want to organize the content from simple to complex, according to issues, or in a timeline (e.g., from the past to the present and then to the future). No matter what organizing method you choose, the following adage provides a good overview of the presentation: Tell them what you are going to say, say it, and then tell them what you have said. In your planning of the presentation, prepare an outline that helps you to organize your content so that your presentation proceeds logically and with clear connections between ideas and thoughts.

4. How can I begin my presentation in a way that grabs the audience's attention?

First, use the course title to capture the audience's attention and arouse curiosity. One presentation on work relations was entitled, "What to Do If Your Boss Is Inebriated, Inept, or Insane." The event organizers said that the presentation was completely booked within one day.

Next, come to the room early (at least 15 minutes before the presentation is scheduled to begin). Use that time to meet people as they enter the room. I often find that my conversations with members of the audience immediately before the presentation can be quite useful when I actually give the presentation. In addition, I often can affirm people's contributions and experience by referring to a prepresentation interaction (e.g., "As George was saying right before the presentation, many of you have dealt with this problem in creative ways.").

It is often helpful to begin presentations with a story or statement that evokes an emotional or startled response from the audience. For example, I often begin presentations about teaching by asking people in the audience to reflect on their experiences with teachers who have had a significant influence in their lives. You can also begin by sharing a startling statistic or newspaper headline (e.g., "Did you know that 1 of every 9 women in this country have been diagnosed with breast cancer?") or by posing a provocative question (e.g., "If we are truly in the era of social and health reform, why are there more people than ever before who are illiterate, imprisoned, and institutionalized?").

5. How can a shy or reserved person entertain an audience?

Attending a presentation by a charismatic performer is often an entertaining experience. But you do not need to be a gifted actor like Robin Williams or Elizabeth Taylor to present well. An excellent performer can be a terrible presenter if he or she does not address the audience's needs or does not know the subject matter. However, you can learn from performers who are effective presenters. They vary their voice tone from time to time; sometimes they are loud, sometimes they are soft. They do not stand in one spot; they move around the room or stage. They laugh often, sometimes at themselves. They use body language to convey important content. They look individual members of the audience in the eye and refer to them in a personal manner (e.g., "I noticed the man with the blue shirt nodding. Sir, tell us about that. Why did you nod?"). They often use personal and other stories that are funny or tragic to make a point. They engage their audience.

6. What can I do to eliminate stage fright when I present to an audience?

Stage fright is a common concern among presenters of all kinds, even musicians, because they want to do a good job but are aware that they may fail and be judged as incompetent. Below are a few strategies that have proven effective in minimizing performance anxiety.

- Prepare for the presentation until you feel that you know it so well that you do not need notes. Preparation instills a sense of control and gives you additional confidence.
- Focus on what the audience is experiencing and learning rather than on how you are performing.
- Prepare yourself emotionally for the presentation. Visualize yourself as presenting with confidence and the audience as enthusiastic. Dress in a way that you feel comfortable but competent. Do exercise or meditation immediately before the presentation if either helps you to feel calm.
- Be yourself. Use your natural speech patterns and mannerisms. If you are not naturally gregarious and charismatic, do not try to be so in a presentation.
- If your mouth dries up when you are nervous, place a glass of water near you. When your mouth is dry, smile at the audience and take a drink. Remember that pauses are helpful in presentations because they give you and the audience time to collect your thoughts.

7. How should I present the content?

The nature of the presentation and the teaching methods that you use depend on the following factors:

- **Your abilities and interests.** Ask yourself, "What are my skills as a presenter? Why did the event organizers invite me to speak? With what teaching strategies am I most comfortable? What teaching strategies would I like to explore?" It is a good general rule, particularly when you are to give presentations to audiences with whom you do not have a longstanding relationship, to stick with teaching strategies that you know best.
- **The nature of audience members and their needs and interests.** In preparing for the presentation, ask yourself, "How much do they know about the topic? What are they hoping to get out of the presentation? What stories and experiences might they come with that I can use to engage them in the presentation? How might their past experiences with the topic, the event organizers, or myself affect their response to the presentation?" You also may want to ask about how the audience traditionally learns new content. For example, if a group of people are used to attending a monthly lecture in which they remain passive, they may be unwilling to entertain teaching strategies that require active involvement, such as participating in a role play.
- **Your goals.** Some content is not appropriate to certain teaching methods. Lecture works well if you want to present facts, but a case study may be better if your aim is to develop the audience's problem-solving skills. In addition, your tone depends on what you are teaching and the audience's reaction. In general, unless you are delivering a presentation about a very serious topic, such as a funeral eulogy, humor works well if used respectfully and judiciously.
- **The nature of the setting.** Some teaching strategies are not applicable in certain rooms because of the size, lighting, and capability for specific audiovisual equipment or teaching strategies. For example, small group discussion probably would be awkward in lecture halls with immovable seats in vertical rows.

8. How should I use audiovisual aids?

If you are going to use audiovisual media, such as slides, make sure that the equipment is operational and practice working the equipment before you give the presentation. Each audiovisual aid has advantages and disadvantages. For example, overhead transparencies are relatively inexpensive and can be substituted easily, even right before the presentation. However, presenters often block the screen because of their position behind the overhead projector. Slides are clear and colorful and can be operated by remote control, but they are expensive and take time to develop. The recent technology of LCD/laptop projections for computer presentations, such as PowerPoint, are clear, easy to animate, and relatively inexpensive. However, LCD projectors and laptops are not available in all facilities, and some rooms are too small for effective projection of presentations (see Chapter 16 for more about computer use in education). Whatever you choose to use, keep the following principles in mind:

- Stick to one or, at the most, two technologies. Presenters who use many different audiovisual media spend a lot of time and energy jumping from machine to machine and usually distract the audience from the actual presentation
- Whenever the audience looks at a screen, attention is diverted away from what you are saying. Consequently, if you are speaking while a slide or overhead is projected on a screen, the audience will not hear much of what you are saying. Make sure that you have only significant points or headings on the slide or overhead and that each slide or overhead contains no more than 5–8 lines of print. Try not to speak when a slide or overhead is on the screen. Switch off the projector before you resume speaking.
- Make sure everyone in the room can see the material. Light printing on dark backgrounds works best for slides, but the opposite is true for overheads. Before the presentation, sit in various chairs throughout the room to assess visibility. The font should be large enough to be seen by everyone in the room (usually 32 points).

- Ask a colleague to preview all slides and overheads for typos. Typographical and spelling errors give the message that you do not care about the audience and that you are sloppy.

9. How can I sustain the audience's interest throughout the presentation?

According to Small's Attention, Relevance, Confidence, and Satisfaction (ARCS) Model of Motivational Design,[7] a presenter needs to sustain listeners' interest and curiosity, to make the presentation relevant and satisfying, and to instill confidence in order for listeners to be attentive to the presentation and motivated to learn from it. The table identifies questions that you can use to plan your presentation according to the ARCS model. You can sustain attention by providing surprise during your presentation or deliberately injecting some uncertainty or conflict. For example, you may present one situation from the perspective of two people, such as a nurse and a patient, to demonstrate opposing views. One cautionary note: while having a herd of elephants walk into the room during a presentation may be surprising and catch people's attention, if you cannot make a connection between the elephants and what you are presenting, neither will your audience. You also can ask questions at certain points in the presentation or invite the audience to find the flaws in your arguments to perk their interest.

Another strategy that fosters people's confidence is to tell them that mastering the content of the presentation is a matter of effort, not ability. Many presenters make the mistake of implying that they are experts because of their intelligence. People in the audience who lack confidence in their ability may respond by admiring the presenter but feeling that the content is too difficult. It is better to make a comment such as, "This may seem difficult at first, but I have found that if people learn a few tricks, they are able to do it. I am going to teach you those tricks today." Lastly, you need to make the presentation relevant to the learner's needs, interests, and goals. Learners are more likely to feel satisfied at the end of your presentation if they know what they have learned, believe it to be valuable in their lives, and have something tangible, such as guidelines, that can help them apply the content.

Self-evaluation of Presentations According to the ARCS Model

DIMENSION	QUESTIONS TO ASK
Attention	Are my teaching materials, such as overheads and handouts, eye-catching? How can I inject some unpredictability, conflict, or surprise into the presentation? How can I vary the ways in which I present information? What questions or projects can I use to pose problems or paradoxes?
Relevance	How can I make clear how the learners will use the content in their work or personal lives? How can I make clear how the content will relate to what learners already know? What examples can I use to relate the material to what learners already know? What language and terminology is appropriate to the learners' level of understanding about the topic? Have I planned to ask the learners to provide examples from their own experience?
Confidence	Is the sequence of information logical? How can I make the content simple enough for the audience's understanding but challenging enough for learners' needs? How can I link their success in applying the content to their lives with effort rather than ability? How can I provide formulas or step-by-step guidelines to assist the audience in applying the content to their lives?
Satisfaction	How will I give credit and recognition to the learners when appropriate, such as recognizing the quality of their participation in class discussions How can I provide ways for learners to assess their own learning, such as pre- and postpresentation testing? How can I provide feedback about questions, ideas, and comments that learners share in the presentation?

10. What can I do to project my voice if I am soft-spoken?

You can use microphones, but they are not always available. Your ordinary conversation voice needs to be a little louder and slower when you are delivering a presentation. A good way of judging how much louder and slower your speech needs to be is to ask a friend to listen to your presentation before you give it, preferably in the same room in which the presentation will take place. Ask the person to sit in various parts of the room to determine whether you can be heard in all areas. Another technique is to let the audience know that you have struggled with projection and to ask them to indicate when they cannot hear you (e.g., "I have a soft voice and sometimes people at the back of the room can't hear me. Can I ask you to raise your hand if you are having trouble hearing me?").

11. What can I do to make the presentation relevant to the audience if I do not know much about them beforehand?

At times when you are asked to give a presentation to a group with whom you have little prior experience. A common example is when a community organization asks you to give a presentation on a particular subject, but you know little about the organization and its members. I have learned over the years always to ask the event planners detailed questions about who will be there and what their needs, interests, and prior experience are likely to be. On one occasion a colleague gave a presentation to an organization of family caregivers of people with severe brain injury. She assumed that only family members would be in attendance. She planned an elaborate slide show to accompany her presentation. Half the audience were people who had survived a brain injury. They became increasingly agitated during the slide presentation because of the overstimulation of colors and lights, and several started yelling and running around the room.

Sometimes you cannot be sure who will come to a presentation because the invitation has been extended to a broad range of people, such as the staff of a hospital. If members of the audience have been required to indicate their attendance in advance, you can request that event organizers ask people to respond with information about their area of work, level of education, and discipline as well as what they consider their top three issues or content areas (see below for an example). You also can request people to give this information immediately before the presentation begins. In this case, however, your agenda has to be flexible enough to permit you to adapt it to the audience's responses. You can quickly tabulate (or ask an event organizer to do so) the responses and say to the audience, "Thank you for completing the form. Your responses indicate that those who are here today come from a range of disciplines and have a variety of experience with and knowledge about today's topic." You can give a general overview of the results and then obtain the audience's views about how to proceed. For example, "There was general agreement that you would like to focus on issues 1 and 6, but the nurses wanted us to talk about issue 3 and the respiratory therapists felt they would like to concentrate on issue 8. How about we begin with issues 1 and 6 and then spend at least 10 minutes each on both 3 and 8? That way we will have some time to discuss any other issues, including any that are not on this list."

Sample Form to Assess Audience's Needs

I am scheduled to present a one-hour session on Critical Thinking in the Workplace on ______ (date/time) at ____________ (location). I may not have had the occasion to meet you before, and I would like to be sure that this presentation meets your needs. Please take a minute to answer these few questions about yourself and what you would like or need in the presentations.

Workplace

Agency: ______________________________

Department or Unit ______________________

Position ______________________________

Please indicate what you would most like to hear about in this presentation by identifying you top three choices. Please number them from 1 (top choice) to 3 (third choice).

Theories of critical thinking ____

Definitions of critical thinking ____

Continued on following page

Critical thinking frameworks ____
Manifestations of critical thinking ____
Challenges in fostering critical thinking ____
Strategies to foster critical thinking ____
Outcomes of critical thinking ____
Other (please indicate a topic that you would like to hear about that is not on this list and its importance to you) ______________________________ (topic) ____ (number).

12. What can I do to structure my presentation so that it is within the allotted time?

Whatever you do when you find yourself either running out of time or finishing way before the allotted time, do not change your pace to make up for it. Speeding up to get through your presentation will accomplish nothing. Alternative strategies include the following:

1. During preparation, you need to identify your "take-home message," one or two sentences that summarize the essence of the presentation. Plan the presentation in 5- to 10-minute blocks with one main idea or point in each block. The take-home message should be in the first, middle, and last block. If time is running out, you can choose to eliminate anything but take-home message blocks.

2. Budget your time for each block. When you are giving the presentation, keep a watch or clock nearby. Stay as close to this budget as possible, but know that you can eliminate blocks if necessary. If you have a tendency to finish your presentation before the allotted time, you can develop additional blocks to be inserted if you find that a lot of time is left and you are nearing your conclusion. Lastly, do not forget to allow time for questions, comments, and sharing by the audience. A rule of thumb is to count on at least 20% of the allotted time for the audience's contributions.

13. What should I do if in the middle of my presentation I lose my concentration and cannot remember what I should say?

This experience is frightening and embarrassing. The more you look at the sea of faces in the audience, the more anxious you tend to be. The strategies to recover and continue the presentation involve giving yourself space to think. First of all, say something about it to the audience, such as, "Excuse me. I was carried away by Joe's story and I have lost my train of thought. I need to look at my notes for a second." This strategy accomplishes a number of goals. It tells the audience that you are human and not afraid to admit it. It also gives the audience a few minutes to think about what you have been saying in the presentation. It gives you permission to take a few seconds to look away from the audience to figure out how you are going to recover. You can also take a few deep breaths to help you to relax. If in a few seconds you are unable to remember what you were going to say and there are no cues in your notes, turn to the audience and say that you will return to the point later.

14. How should I end the presentation?

An effective conclusion ties up any loose ends and reviews what has been said in the presentation, leaving the audience wanting more. It should be as powerful and provocative as your opening statement. A rule of thumb is to leave them thinking about the topic. For example, end with a statement such as, "All that we have had time for today is to briefly explore the issues pertaining to medication errors. It's a little like putting your toe into the ocean and saying you now can identify all the fish that live there. However, perhaps this introduction will encourage you to explore this subject in greater depth in the future."

15. How can I best handle questions from the audience?

Listen carefully to the question and write a few notes if it is complicated. Thank the person for the question. Be careful about giving positive comments about questions (e.g., "That is such an interesting question") because if you fail to make similar comments about all questions that arise, others may be offended or think that their questions are unsatisfactory. Rephrase the question (e.g., "Correct me if I am wrong, but what I heard you say was __________"). Repeating the question allows you to collect your thoughts about the answer and enables audience members who may not have heard the question the first time to hear it again. If you do not know the answer, admit it and ask if anyone in the audience has anything to offer. If no one in the audience knows the answer, ask the person who asked the question for his or her name, e-mail address, or telephone number and agree to get back with the answer in a specified time.

16. How do I obtain feedback about my presentation skills?

There are a number of ways. One common way is to hand everyone in the audience a short piece of paper at the beginning of the presentation. You should explain that you would like to know your strengths and limitations as a presenter so that you can continue to grow. You would like them to spend two minutes at the end of this session answering these questions: (1) What grade would you give this presentation (from F to A+)? and (2) Why did you give this grade? The simpler you make the feedback tool, the more likely it is that people will complete it. In addition, you can ask colleagues to attend the session and assess your presentation on specific criteria (e.g., "I have always had trouble with the pacing of my presentations. Could you observe how I do in this regard?"). This is the most effective method if you trust and respect the colleague's opinion and know that he or she will be honest and help you to resolve any difficulties that you encounter in the presentation. Another evaluative technique is to videotape yourself and to observe your presentation after you deliver it. Abernathy[1] includes a self-evaluation checklist that you can use to critique yourself.

BIBLIOGRAPHY

1. Abernathy DJ: Presentation tips from the pros. Train Devel 53:19–26, 1999.
2. Andrica DC: Executive development: Making good oral presentations. Nurs Econ 17:272, 1999.
3. Bender PU: Secrets of Power Presentations. Toronto, WEBCOM, 2000.
4. Evans ML: Polished, professional presentation: Unlocking the design elements. J Contin Educ Nurs 31:213–218, 2000.
5. Farr JV: Developing your oral communication skills. J Manage Engineer 16:6, 2000.
6. Noreiko P: Taking the fear out of presentations. Occup Health 47:312–315, 1995.
7. Small R: Motivation in Instructional Design. Washington, DC, ERIC Clearinghouse on Information and Technology (ED409895), 1997.

15. CREATIVE TEACHING STRATEGIES

Kristen L. O'Shea, MS, RN

1. Why is choice of strategy so important?

As a nursing staff development educator, your job is to help make the information that you present come alive for the nurses and clinical staff. It is no longer acceptable to stand up and lecture, giving copious amounts of information. Good teachers understand that what it takes to effect learning is more important than teaching itself. Your goals are to create an environment that is conducive to learning and to plan a variety of activities that enhance that learning process. What you know about adult learning helps you to understand why a variety of teaching strategies is necessary to help nurses learn. Adults learn best if (1) the information is relevant to their situation; (2) individual differences are taken into account; and (3) the learners are actively involved in the learning process (see Chapter 10). Using a variety of teaching strategies can help to enhance learning for adults.

2. How do I begin?

Begin with your objectives. After you have written clear, measurable objectives, you should ask yourself, "How can we get to these objectives?" Brainstorm or find ideas in activity books. Think of all of the possible ways in which you can get your content across to the group that you are teaching.

3. What is the best way to teach nurses?

There is no single best way to teach nurses. There are many ways to facilitate involvement with the material and appeal to learning styles. You must take into consideration many factors.

Educator factors

- Length of time you have to teach
- Your level of experience and comfort with teaching strategies
- Amount of money that you have
- Length of time you have for preparation
- Topic

Participant factors

- How well the participants know one another (including comfort level)
- Learning style(s)
- Degree to which participants are familiar with the topic

4. When should I lecture?

I would like to say, "You should never lecture." To me, lecturing represents a dependent and inactive process. However, it is important to understand that at times lecture may be necessary, and it is up to you to use lecture in conjunction with other methods to enhance learning.

Time constraints and large numbers of participants often limit your ability to use more interactive techniques. Many of the techniques covered below take time to do well, particularly if you have a large group. In addition, it is often necessary to lecture when you are providing a large amount of new information. In all of these cases, take measures to enhance your lecture with visual aids and opportunities for audience participation and interaction.

5. How can I jazz up my lecture?

At a minimum, you must use lots of visual aids. Visual aids help to engage the visual learner. Auditory learners may do well by listening to a lecture, but visual learners need the added boost of well-designed visual aids to maintain their attention and to paint a picture. This approach helps to ensure that you cover the main points with them. Consider a variety of visuals and illustrations.

In addition, handouts help to reinforce your spoken word and to keep visual and kinesthetic learners on task. One suggestion is to provide handouts with the important points in print. Omit key words so that participants need to interact with the material by filling in the blanks. Handouts should include an outline of the material that you cover, copies of illustrations or graphs, and additional resources and references.

Asking questions is another simple method to engage the participants in the lecture. Open-ended questions such as "Can you give an example of this?" or "What application of this have you seen on your area?" provide learners with an opportunity to apply information to their own experiences and help others who may be struggling with applicability in their own setting.

Use of stories and anecdotes also helps to maintain interest. Participants often tell me that they remember the content because of the story that I told. However, you should carefully plan your stories to ensure that they are relevant and that you do not forget key information in the heat of the moment. The same goes for demonstrations—plan them carefully. They can have a great impact in helping people remember what you were lecturing about.

6. What should I *not* do when I lecture?

Cooper[1] lists several "Lecture Don'ts" that you need to keep in mind:

- Never write out your lecture and read it. This method is dull, dull, dull.
- Do not include too much information. Focus on your objectives.
- Never talk longer than 2 hours without a break. I try to intersperse questions and stories every 8–10 minutes to break the pace and offer a break every 1½–2 hours. Try stand-up breaks when you see the group (or yourself) fading.
- Avoid distracting mannerisms or repetitive phrases. Ask your colleagues to help identify examples in your presentation. If you play with markers, make an effort to put them down. If you jingle the change in your pocket, take it out. If you say "ummmm" or "you know," make conscious efforts to take a pause as you feel it coming out. A pause is better than an "ummmm."
- Never lecture or preach. Use a conversational tone.

7. How do I go about choosing a strategy to use?

This question is not as easy to answer as it sounds. Because the process is individual to your situation, it will take some research and experimentation to find the right mix for you. In general, you should always be on the look-out for new approaches. Collect strategies. Go to conferences, and sit in on your colleagues' sessions to see what works. You should experiment with new strategies. Use books to identify possible games and activities. There is a wealth of resources that can help you. Part of the fun is finding the mix that works for you. This chapter identifies potential strategies for you to use.

8. What strategies should I always use?

1. **Have an icebreaker activity, or, at minimum, conduct introductions to set a tone.** Try to show that you and the participants are going to have fun and that this is a safe environment. Many books contain icebreakers. An icebreaker is any activity that helps others get to know one another. You should develop a file of icebreakers that you like to use. Examples include the following:

- All participants are asked to write three truths and one lie about themselves on 3 × 5 card and to read them to group. The group decides which is the lie. As an alternative, participants pass their cards to the instructor, who reads them aloud. Participants decide whose card it is and then which statement is the lie.
- Ask participants to pick a television show, actor/actress, or occupation with which they identify and tell the group why.
- Create a list of interests or characteristics, and ask members of the group to get the signatures of other members who share that characteristic (e.g., drives a red car, is married to a lawyer, has a dog, likes anchovies on pizza). Give participants 10 minutes to meet as many people as possible.
- Have the group split into dyads (suggest that they pair with someone whom they have not met before), and ask each member of the dyad to introduce his or her partner.

2. **Establish the group's expectations.** You want to know why they are present. For example, use large group discussion and ask volunteers to help generate a list of reasons for their attendance

and issues that they would like to cover during the session. Post the list in the front of the room so that you can be sure to cover the topics in which the group is interested. There are many reasons for doing an activity such as this. First, you are interested in barriers to learning. In many cases, participants give an answer such as "I don't know. My manager told me to come." Such answers are important to know, because your job is to convince the participants that you have something to share that is of importance (relevance) to them. Secondly, it is important that you know exactly what people need to know. Obviously, you have planned material for your presentation based on a "need"; however, you must be sure that you meet the participants' perceived current needs. Perhaps you are teaching a charge nurse course, and a participant has just experienced a conflict that needs to be addressed. By identifying participants' expectations, you are able to keep your content relevant. If you are unable to cover content that participants have identified, you need to direct them to a source of information. This approach sends another important message: you care about what they want to know.

3. **Plan your conclusion carefully.** The conclusion is your opportunity to emphasize the key points one last time. This important step helps to tie everything together, particularly if you have chosen a variety of strategies. Sometimes when participants are involved in games or small group work, they do not get the "ah-hah" until you take the time to pull it altogether.

9. Why should I use games?

- To promote active participation
- To help review and promote retention of knowledge (games are not intended to present new information)
- To enhance group interaction and teamwork
- To promote creative thinking
- To apply theory to real-life experiences
- In some cases, to allow players to practice in a simulated environment without fear of serious consequences.

10. Why do games have a bad reputation among some people?

For some people, it is hard to imagine that you can have fun and learn at the same time. In some education circles, gaming is not seen as a serious educational tool. In addition, games that are not well planned are seen as a waste of time or fail to make their point.

Games, however, can be a highly effective tool when they are appropriate to the topic and well planned. Adult learners are competitive. Games certainly increase the interaction of participants with the content. Finally, people have fun playing games—and learning is enhanced when participants are having fun. Retention may be increased up to 90% when a game is used effectively.[2]

11. What games should I use?

A game can be created to fit almost any content. For subject-specific content, it is possible to use any of the common popular game formats and, with time, to create a game that reinforces your content. Game boards can be created out of cardboard or display boards. Velcro works nicely to attach game pieces or clues to fabric display boards. It is also possible to purchase software that allows you to create games and run them in a classroom with use of an LCD panel (see Chapter 14). Possibilities include the following:

- Name That ______ (body part, system, rhythm, diagnosis)
- Trivial Pursuit (for obstetrics, emergency departments, pediatrics)
- Who Wants to Be a Millionaire? (any topic)
- Jeopardy (advanced cardiac life support, pharmacology, oncology)
- Find What's Wrong (safety issues)
- Family Feud (for intensive care unit; top complications of ________)
- Candy Land (e.g., for obstetrics; a decision-making game for placement of patients when a new mother/baby unit is opened)
- Wheel of Fortune (any topic)
- The Price Is Right (reinforce fiscal responsibility in staff with cost of supplies)
- Friday Night in the ER (a decision-making game)

Games should have prizes. Adults are highly competitive when prizes are awarded. Prizes can be simple and practical (e.g., pens, Post-It notes, box of tissues), fun (e.g., clown nose, magic wand, small game or gadget), edible (e.g., candy bars or gum), or applicable to the game (a symbol from the game, such as a fire hat for the person who knows the most about fire safety or a million dollars in fake money). Start a drawer in which you collect possible prizes. You may see them at a convention or on a Saturday trip to Wal-Mart. When you see something that may work as a prize, buy it. Taking that step encourages you to try a game in your next class.

12. Do people definitely hate role-plays?

Yes and no. The problem with role-plays is that participants feel performance pressure. Sometimes inadequate leadership and planning are provided. Role-plays are complex. But instructors can create role-play scenarios in which the participants can "practice" skills that they learn in a safe environment. Role-plays should be used when adequate time has been given to the development of a secure learning environment. In addition, participants must be given enough information to complete the role-play in order for it to be successful.

13. What process should I use in developing a role-play or case study?

You must carefully select a pertinent issue. In the case of role-play, the topics usually involve human dynamics or problem-solving. With a case study, you are trying to promote critical thinking and decision-making. Next, develop an incident or situation. Write down the details about this incident. You need to give enough detail for the participants to be able to carry out the role-play and meet the objectives of the activity. Nothing is worse than participating in a role-play when you do not know what to do. Be sure that you clearly communicate the objectives of the exercise.

You also need to plan how you are going to set up the participants. Set the size of the groups. For example, you may decide that two people will role-play a scenario and one person will be an observer. This method is a little less intimidating than performing a role-play in front of an entire group. You should provide an evaluation tool so that the observer knows what he or she is looking for.

You need to decide how the groups will be formed. If you have a mix of staff you may want oncology nurses together, ICU nurses together, and so on. Or you may want to mix the groups a bit and have a day-shift nurse with a night-shift nurse.

Lastly, determine the time that you are going to allow for the activity. Careful planning of all these details ahead of time helps to make your activity a success.

14. List examples of other activities that I can try.

- Field trips to hospital departments or pharmaceutical companies
- Small group discussions
- Large group discussions
- Debates
- Video clips
- Clinical lab simulation
- Interpersonal simulation activities
- Crossword puzzles
- Brain teasers
- Skits
- Projects
- Expert panels
- Patient testimonials
- Storytelling
- Brainstorming
- Group care planning
- Articles
- Computer-assisted instruction

15. What resources are available to help me add fun to learning activities?

You should begin to collect books of activities and games. A wide range of books contain detailed descriptions of games that can be used for all sorts of educational session.[2,6–9] Many nurse educators are familiar with a nurse-operated company by the name of Tool Thyme for Trainers, which carries creative products and books.[2] The company can be reached at www.tooltrainers.com. Another source of creative tips is Bob Pike's site: www.creativetraining tech.com. The following websites also are fun to use:

- www.quia.com (for game development)
- www.puzzlemaker.com (for design of various puzzles, such as crossword, word search)

16. Is humor an effective instructional strategy?

Absolutely. A great deal of evidence shows that humor is a great strategy to promote learning. As Klein said, "To get 'em listening, get 'em laughing."[3] You need to plan in advance how to incorporate humor into your educational session. You may try to add jokes, funny skits, or stories and comics to your lectures. I keep a folder in my closest desk drawer where I slip medical comics and jokes for future use. Numerous books contain medical humor as well. *Medicalese: A Humorous Medical Dictionary* is available through AVIAN-Cetacean Press.

Music is another way to introduce humor into your lecture. Various humorous songs on the market can spice up your lecture. Short humorous video clips also provide examples of fun. For example, when teaching content on labor and delivery, I have used clips from sit-com versions of labor and delivery (Murphy Brown's labor is my favorite).

17. What educational options are available for nurses who cannot leave the floor?

Educators need to create ways to support the education of busy staff in clinical areas. It is important to work with the nurse managers in planning staff education. If you are planning an all-day program, plenty of notice must be given so that the schedule can allow some of the staff to attend.

Unless time-off is scheduled for education, staff are usually unable to leave the busy clinical areas. Below are some ideas to start your creative juices flowing:

- Consider having short 10-minute roving rounds on a highly specific topic.
- Post information about a topic on the staff bulletin board in an attractive manner, or, better yet, post it on the back of the bathroom door and call it "Potty Training."
- Show short videos to staff with tests.
- Include short topics in staff meetings.
- Investigate computer options that can be completed in short periods.
- Use self-learning packets.
- Use on-the-unit experts or superusers.

The reality is that staff are no longer able to "come to us." Instead, educators must develop ways to get education to the staff.

18. What is a superuser?

A superuser is someone who has been specially trained to teach others about a new piece of equipment or to support a new computer application after a computer-based training program has been completed. Superusers are highly effective educational tools, particularly because it is possible to support people in their clinical areas seven days per week. They are particularly helpful in educating evening and night-shift staff. The time used for mentoring superusers to provide education to a small core group during working hours is time well spent. Examples of areas in which superusers can be trained for educational purposes:

- Clinical computer applications
- New IV pump
- Upgrades in systems or equipment
- New forms for documentation

19. What should I keep in mind when using superusers to provide education or training?

- Make sure that superusers know the scope of what they are expected to do.
- Provide written objectives and outlines.
- Provide superusers with plenty of trouble-shooting information and resources.
- Ensure that there are enough superusers in each area. (One suggestion is to have enough superusers available for each shift of the weekend. If the unit is staffed with 12-hour shifts every third weekend, have a minimum of six superusers.)
- Provide support and recognition of superusers during the implementation of the new equipment or application.

20. What are self-learning modules?

Self-learning modules are packets of materials designed to allow independent study of a specific topic. Other terms include self-learning packets (SLPs), self-paced modules, and independent study units.

21. What are the benefits of SLPs?

- SLPs are available 24 hours per day.
- SLPs are portable.
- Learners can pursue information that is needed or relevant.
- SLPs involve the learner in the educational process and provide self-direction and individual responsibility.
- The learner can be interrupted and then resume as able.
- SLPs can be used to provide didactic information, allowing the educator to tackle more in-depth educational needs or topics that require interpersonal contact.
- SLPs are a means of providing consistent education to large groups of students who may not be able to leave the clinical areas for a class.
- SLPs provide great flexibility for part-time or as-needed staff.

22. How do I go about creating an SLP?

Like any classroom offering, an SLP starts with the development of measurable objectives to meet a need. Most SLPs contain objectives, directions for use, a list of learning activities, content that is visually pleasant and easily readable, a posttest, and a learner evaluation of the SLP. Length of the SLP depends on the topic, but it is important to consider the amount of time that the staff at your hospital is willing to put into a self-learning packet. I try to keep the length to about 1 hour's worth of content, including the post-test and evaluation. It is possible to use a variety of visual aids as part of the SLP. Participants can be asked to watch a video and then take a posttest in the form of a crossword puzzle. It is quite possible to make SLPs creative and fun.

23. Expert nurses often teach by reading their notes to the class. How can I help them to become better teachers?

Consider a presenter workshop. Not everyone has experience with teaching a class. Many expert nurses are nervous, have had no time for preparation, and model "lectures" that they received in nursing school. You have an obligation to help them enhance their presentation skills. The content is very important to learners in the course. Consider choosing topics from the following list to develop a course for nurses who educate others:

- Presentation skills
- Adult learning theory
- Learner diversity
- Creative teaching strategies
- Use of computer applications (e.g., PowerPoint)
- Use of audiovisual equipment
- Evaluation of learning

In addition, content from Chapters 10–15 may be useful

24. Give examples of how creative strategies can be incorporated into a lesson about the renal system.

The following lesson was developed by Linda Caputi, MSN, EdD, Professor of Nursing at College of DuPage in Glen Ellyn, Illinois:

To begin the lecture, I play a song titled "Doin' the Incontinence Rag" by Too Live Nurse (lyrics by Robert Diskin, RN; music by Edward Fiebke, RN; used with permisison from Muse-Med Inc.). I distribute copies of the lyrics so that students can sing along. Below are two stanzas:

There's a new dance sensation,
That's flooding the nation.
Done by nurses from Maine to L.A.
And we sing all the louder,
As we wash, wipe and powder,
And our patients stay dry all the day,
All the day.

Always cause for celebration,
When you catch that micturation,
It really blows your I & Os,
When you're doing the incontinence rag.
Gosh, oh gee, and holy, moly,
Can I please insert a Foley.
It's Depends, or Attends,
When you're doing the incontinence rag.

This song encourages laughter, relaxes the students, and puts them in a "urinary" mindset. It is highly effective in meeting all three of these objectives.

The handout packet begins with a one-page outline of the lecture. On this page is a cartoon of a nurse in a physician's office with the sign "Urinary Clinic." The nurse is on the phone and is saying, "Can you hold?" A review of this outline gives the students an overview of the 2½-hour session. We then have our first drawing with subsequent drawings every 30 minutes.

The lecture begins with overhead transparencies containing cartoons. These transparencies are included in the students' lecture packet. Students follow through each page, adding notes as needed. Students say that this lecture packet helps them focus on what I am saying rather than frantically writing down every word.

As I discuss the normal physiology of the kidneys I project selected parts of the software program *The PhysWhiz: The Renal System*. This program contains graphics and animation that demonstrate visually what I am explaining. Many of the screens have additional thinking questions or practice items that engage students' participation. They are helpful in getting the students to think actively about what I am saying rather than to listen passively.

Whenever possible, I challenge students with a hinky-pinky. A hinky-pinky is a humorous, rhyming explanation of a situation. Examples include the following:

Defintion: What a urologist spends his/her day doing

Answer: Curin' urine

Definition: An overdistended urinary drainage bag

Answer: A roly-poly Foley

A 15-minute break is provided after the first hour. Soft, relaxing music is played during the break for students who remain in the room and while students are returning from break. To start the session after break, I present *The Top 10 Reasons to Be Thankful We Have Kidneys*:

10. Without them, a couple of cans of pop and we'd explode.

9. Kidneys promote family harmony. Better be nice to your siblings; some day you may need one of their kidneys.

8. Dialysis Rotation Observation Day: stress-free clinical day

7. To provide the opportunity to relate nursing skills to culture, such as inserting a 16-French Foley catheter

6. Without kidneys, what would you call kidney bean salad?

5. Studying the renal system gives another chance to figure out all that electrolyte stuff.

4. Without kidneys and the formation of urine, your lecture would go on and on for the full 2½ hours. Kidneys mean a potty break!

3. Kidneys provide the opportunity to use the word *micturate*.

2. Using the restroom to micturate provides some challenges in your life, such as how to use those dryers. Instructions: Wash hands; rub vigorously under dryer; wipe hands on pants.

1. Without kidneys we would look like this:

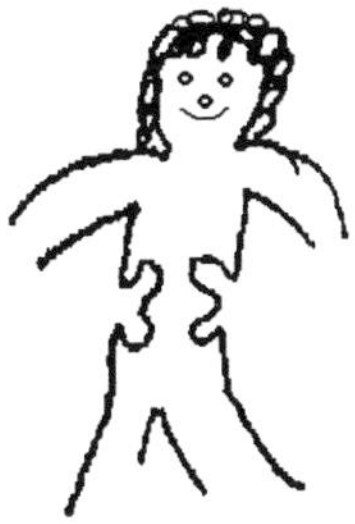

The top 10 list helps increase student endorphin levels through laughter. The lecture then continues through the packet, which incorporates many cartoons to keep the endorphin levels high.

In addition, as I discuss various pathologic conditions, I show a slide of diseased tissue to demonstrate the condition. I intersperse the slides throughout the lecture. This technique is more helpful than showing all of the slides at the end of the lecture.

Finally, when the lecture is over, I distribute a rap that incorporates many of the topics discussed in the class:

The Renal Rap

Now that it's test time,
Let's review.
Bladder, ureters,
And kidneys, too.

Let's start with the nephron,
That's where the action's at.
125 mLs a minute,
Can't beat that!

The blood pH is dropping,
The kidneys play a part.
Secrete that extra hydrogen,
Before acidosis even starts.

How are the kidneys working?
Let's check out the labs today.
We could look at the BUN,
But creatinine's a better way.

Now that it's test time,
Let's review.
Bladder, ureters,
And kidneys, too.

Pathologies can happen,
In every part of the urinary tract.
Like urinary tract infection,
E. coli knows about that!

Let's eradicate those bugs,
Get a C & S for UT's sake.
Culture to see what's growing,
Sensitivity shows the right drug to take.

Diuretics are helpful drugs,
When too much fluid you retain.
Works on what part of the kidney nephron?
Tubule is the name.

Now that it's test time,
Let's review.
Bladder, ureters,
And kidneys, too.

Acute pyelonephritis
Isn't so cute you say.
Bring on those IV antibiotics,
That'll make it go away.

Oh, my, what a pain!
Stones caught in the tract.
Better strain all that urine,
Diet changes so they don't come back!

Remember specific gravity?
What's ARF's affect?
Can't concentrate or dilute,
At 1010 spec grav gets fixed.

Now that it's test time,
Let's review.
Bladder, ureters,
And kidneys, too.

CRF, that's the path,
That's really most severe.
Some of the things that can go wrong,
Is what you're about to hear.

Phosphate really takes to task,
All the calcium in the bones.
Mealtime aluminum hydroxide,
Then it'll leave the calcium alone.

The skin is so very itchy,
Makes him angry and cross.
Look closer and you'll see,
Crystals of uremic frost!

Now that it's test time,
Let's review.
Bladder, ureters,
And kidneys, too.

Tuberculosis you might think,
Is in the lungs for sure.
Did you think it's in the kidney?
Rifampin could be a cure.

Kidney transplants now are common.
Happens every day.
So to not reject that kidney
Cyclosporine on the way!

Now it's almost test time,
That's the end of the review.
My advice is to really study,
And, good luck to you!

BIBLIOGRAPHY

1. Cooper SS: Teaching tips: Some lecturing do's and don'ts. J Contin Educ Nurs 20:140–141, 1989.
2. Deck ML: Instant Teaching Tools for Health Care Educators. St. Louis, Mosby, 1995.
3. Hayes SK, Childress DM: Games galore. J Nurs Staff Devel 16:168–170, 2000.
4. Fuszard B: Innovative Teaching Strategies in Nursing, 2nd ed. Gaithersburg, MD, Aspen, 1995.
5. Klein A: Quotations to Cheer You Up When the World Is Getting You Down. Avenel, NJ, Wings Books, 1994. p 130.
6. Riley JB: Instant Tools for Health Care Teams. St. Louis, Mosby, 1997.
7. Scannell EE, Newstrom JW: Games Trainers Play. New York, McGraw-Hill, 1980.
8. Scannell EE, Newstrom JW: More Games Trainers Play. New York, McGraw-Hill, 1983.
9. Scannell EE, Newstrom JW: Still More Games Trainers Play. New York, McGraw–Hill, 1991.

16. USING COMPUTERS IN EDUCATION

Kenneth R. *Bowman*, RN, MS

Chapter 5, Computer Skills for Educators, discusses several general computer applications that can be used as tools in staff development. This chapter deals with computer applications specifically designed for use as educational material or as tools to manage and document the educational process. Applications for education range from computer-based/browser-based training programs to educational databases called learning management systems (LMSs). Many of these applications are categorized as E-learning.

1. What is E-learning?

E-learning is the next step in the evolutionary process of using computers in education. It is best defined as any instruction that is delivered electronically. This definition includes such methods as computer-based training (CBT), web-based training (WBT), Internet-based training, online courses, and even live Internet broadcasts. E-learning also refers to the systems that manage education and the educational records. The concept of teaching by computer or managing education through the computer is relatively new to staff development. This trend began in health care training around the late 1980s. Today most nursing programs use some form of E-learning as part of their curriculum.

2. Why consider E-learning in staff development?

E-learning is valuable in staff development for various reasons. E-learning can help any staff development department reach its customers (staff members) better by providing training 24 hours per day. CBT, WBT, and Internet-based training can provide education where and when the staff wants to use it. E-learning can be used during periods when floors are quiet or on days when staffing is better than average. To managers, E-learning seems like a positive concept, because it makes productive use of staff downtime. E-learning is also a highly flexible tool for learners, who can take the course at their own pace. Flexibility is an important concept of adult education.

3. Is there a down side to E-learning?

A major issue with E-learning is that many staff members are not comfortable with learning from a computer screen. The population that we are teaching has a mean age of 35 years or older. Many of them are still new to the computer. They may have a computer at home, but do not assume that they are the primary user. Sitting at a computer for long periods does not fit the concept of learning for many staff. Another issue is how management looks at E-learning. Often management considers E-learning as a way to replace staff educators. E-learning can produce a cost savings for an education department, but it never replaces what a live person can do in training a staff member. E-learning can allow a staff educator to reduce time spent on repetitive training programs (e.g., Occupational Safety and Health Administration [OSHA], Joint Commission for the Accreditation of Healthcare Organizations [JCAHO]) and allow the educator to spend more high-quality time with staff members.

4. What other issues are relevant to the use of E-learning?

Technical requirements can make or break the ability to use E-learning effectively. The first step in assessing whether your institution is ready to begin using any of form of E-learning is to find out what hardware and software are available and whether E-learning forms will work with them. Find a good technical advisor for this task. Look to your information systems department for an expert with whom you can feel comfortable. Comfort is important, because it is easy to get lost in technical talk. You need a good interpreter. Do not expect to do an E-learning project alone.

Another important point is to make sure that your staff members are ready for this new direction in learning. Talk with the staff, and, if possible, have staff members as part of the selection committee. Make sure that you have management's support for two reasons: purchasing the software and getting the staff to use it. The process of purchasing the software is a major part of E-learning. The up-front cost of E-learning is quite high. For example, a single program on a CD may cost between $200 and $1000. For a complete system, the minimal investment is $10,000–$20,000. Make sure that you show management staff members the costs and, even more importantly, the benefits that a system provides for your institution. Once the system is in place, management backing is needed to encourage staff use. Managers need to be willing to make the content of your E-learning a mandatory part of employees' educational process.

5. What is computer-based training (CBT)?

CBT is the least technologically intense format of E-learning. CBTs are similar to computer game programs; you purchase them from a vendor and use them directly on your personal computer (PC). CBTs can be purchased from medical publishing companies as individual programs or as sets of programs. An excellent example of a CBT series is the Lippincott William & Wilkins series on critical care nursing. In addition, several small but specialized vendors can supply CBTs for medication math or critical thinking.

Several different types of CBTs are currently available. The simplest are **tutorials**, sometimes called "electronic page turners." Tutorials provide training in the format of text on the screen. The user's only interaction with the program is to click forward or backward, page by page. The tutorial CBT tends to be the least liked by users because of reading from a computer screen. Most users still prefer the written word for reading.

Drill and practice CBTs are excellent tools to teach such concepts as medication math or arterial blood gas analysis. The user completes tasks such as a series of math problems. If mistakes are made, the programs may have the user repeat new problems until a threshold of correctness is met. Drill and practice CBTs can be used as part of competency programs or as remediation for staff members with special issues.

The final form of CBT is the **simulation** program, which provides training by showing the user a complete case scenario. The unique advantage of a simulation is that an inexperienced person can experience a dangerous situation without endangering a real patient. Simulations are also popular because they encourage deeper levels of critical thinking. Critical thinking, one of the most difficult areas to teach, is not normally taught in a classroom; simulations are a possible solution. Simulations are also popular with younger staff members because of their experience with computer gaming from a young age.

6. What technical issues need to be addressed with the use of CBT?

You need to decide whether the program will reside on a single PC or be made available on many computers. Purchasing a CBT does not mean that you can load it on as many PCs as you wish. Each set-up requires a license.

It is possible to set up a CBT so that it can be accessed through a network from a server, but this approach requires a site license. If you consider setting up a network, make sure that the computer systems can handle it. Setting up a CBT on a network requires two items in addition to the PC: a server and the network. The server size depends on how many people will use the CBT at any given time. The more people accessing the software, the larger the server must be. If the server is too small, the system is too slow to use. Make sure that a good information system support person assists you in making this decision. The network is also important to assess before you go ahead with a CBT set up. The network consists of the wires and computers that interconnect the PC and the server. Networks are like pipelines. The smaller the pipe, the less water (or, in the case of the network, information) that can flow through it. The important point to remember is that the network is designed to carry all of the hospital's information—not just the CBT program. A disaster may result if using the educational software slows down the clinical systems; make sure to involve your hospital's network manager in the CBT discussion.

7. What is the difference between CBT and WBT?

Web-based training (WBT) is quite similar to CBT in terms of style and content. WBT comes in the same three designs: tutorials, drill and practice, and simulations. The major difference is how the material is delivered to the user. WBT cannot even be considered if your institution does not have an intranet system. WBT uses web technologies to create and deliver the content to PCs that have access to an intranet system. In addition to having an intranet, a WBT system requires a computer on which to store the programs and the program system. Some companies can provide web-based programs that are already built. The other option is to buy a program that allows you to build your own web-based programs. This option sounds great, until you learn that it takes considerable time to plan and create a web-based program. Be on the lookout for some real improvements in this area.

If you want to create a simple tutorial type of WBT, you may already have a program that can do so. Check your presentation program (PowerPoint or Presentation) to see whether you have a version that can put a presentation into HTML format. HTML is the Internet programming language and can be used to create your presentation on the intranet. If you are considering any type of WBT program, make sure that you are on friendly terms with your intranet web master, who can help you get your system to function from the intranet.

8. Can I use the Internet for training?

Internet-based programs are the newest entry in the staff development field. They are commonly called education portals and are provided by application service providers (ASP). These programs are designed, owned, and sold by ASP companies as a way to provide ongoing education for clinical staff. Most of these companies began by providing continuing medical education for physicians, but since more nurses are using the Internet, they have turned their attention to providing continuing education units (CEUs). If you are in a state where CEUs are required for licensure, Internet-based programs are a convenient way to provide staff education. Many companies also offer programs that meet the requirements for JCAHO or OSHA training.

When you contact ASP companies about training, you will find them more than willing to sell you contracts for staff training. These contracts are typically written in terms of the number of users and the number of programs to which each user will be given access. The total amount determines the cost. Such contracts are typically written in costs per year. If you are considering Internet-based programs, make sure that you shop around. The cost per year can vary greatly from company to company.

Another issue that you will face when using Internet-based programs is hour and wage regulations. If your clinical staff members are still considered hourly employees, allowing them to complete required training from the Internet at home may mean that they need to be compensated for that time. Make sure that you involve a member of the human resources staff when considering this form of training. Lastly, do not forget to include your information systems person in the discussion. If the training is going to be on the Internet and used through the hospital's computers, you must ask information systems whether the Internet system can handle the information traffic. Moving toward Internet-based training may result in an expansion of the Internet system for the hospital.

9. What is the next step in E-learning for staff development?

On-line courses and Internet broadcasts are beginning to take hold in large medical centers as a way to provide training for staff. On-line courses are conducted through the use of a website and e-mail. There are two designs for these types of courses. **Live interactive courses** allow the user to communicate directly with an instructor via Internet video. In **on-demand courses**, users interact with instructors by e-mail. Good examples of on-line courses can be found at most colleges and universities. For the most part, on-line courses have been limited to college level education; however, the concept has potential for staff education.

Another educational tool is the Internet broadcast. Internet broadcasts are lectures or discussion panels that are broadcast via the Internet from a central site to anyone participating. Unlike satellite television programs, Internet broadcasts do not require special hook-ups. The hardware consists of a computer, Internet connection, and usually a speaker phone with an outside line. If you use this format for a group of people, an LCD projector is also needed. When you sign up to participate in a program of this type, you are given a website address. At the time of the program, linking into the website provides you with either the presentation material or actual video of the speaker. The phone is used at this point to call into the site to access the audible portion of the presentation. Most Internet broadcasts still use this method because the audio is much better over the phone than through the computer. This technology will change as Internet audio improves. If you are wondering what kind of Internet broadcasts are available, check the websites for national nursing conferences. Many are now making Internet broadcasts available.

10. How do I track E-learning along with regular training?

This question points to another type of computer software that is highly valuable to staff education—the database. Databases are available in three levels: basic, midlevel, and high-end learning management systems. It is important to start with basic information before we discuss these computer tools.

11. What is a database?

Before discussing the database, the concept of data must be clarified. Data (which is actually the plural of datum) are best viewed as the smallest elements of information that can be put into a file. For staff development, data may include such items as the name, length, and date of the class and who taught it. Even this information can be broken down into smaller pieces of data. The length of a class consists of two elements: the number of minutes or hours and the designation for minutes or hours, depending on which is used. Both elements are separate data. Data must be viewed as the smallest parts of what make up the information that we use. The ability to break data into small parts, store it, and then retrieve it to make it whole again is the foundation of the database.

A database is an application that organizes data. The database allows the data to be accessed, manipulated, updated, and, most importantly, used to create reports. A database starts with a table similar to a spreadsheet. Unlike a spreadsheet, a database works from many tables at one time. Data elements are stored in separate fields in the tables. These fields have their own name and connections to other data. The connection between data is made through the use of a key or key field. The key field is a unique identifier in the database. No two keys can be alike. For example, in a database of employees, each employee may have an employee number. No two employees can have the same number; otherwise, the information becomes jumbled and is of little value. This unique key is used to connect the data fields throughout the tables, thus allowing the user to pull the data back into some form of information.

12. Can I use the Access database for educational records?

Yes. Many different types of databases are currently available. The simplest and cheapest is Microsoft Access, one of the programs included in the Microsoft Office software. This software may already be available to you. Access can be used to create a simple database in which you can keep the names, identifiers, and basic educational records for the staff that you are training. A database of this type can be set up with basic knowledge of the program. It is important to have some understanding of Access before you try and build your first database—not so much because Access is hard to use, but more because it is too easy to create junk information. Before you even begin the process of setting up a simple database such as Access, you must put some thought into what you are going to enter into the database and what you want to get out. Many people forget the second part and thus, end up with information of little value.

It is possible to make a powerful database out of Access, but a person well versed in Access is required take it to that level. On the other hand, it does not require a degree in computer science to achieve high-quality results. If you suspect that you will need to depend on an Access database for your information, it may be wise to take a class in Access before trying to use the program. More advanced classes may be needed as your database begins to grow.

13. Can I purchase rather than build a training database program?

Yes. Basic programs can often meet the needs of a small education department and are available for $500–$1000. These programs are designed to meet only the basic needs of an education department. If you are considering a program in this price range, make sure that you are getting something that is usable for your department. The process of entering information into the system should be easy. Typically there is a data entry screen into which you type information. You should not need to reenter the information multiple times. For example, once you put an employee's name into the database, you should be able to recall him or her to update the information. It is also important that the system provide reports that meet your needs. All training database systems should be able to generate a report that shows who attended a course and when. You also should be able to generate a report that shows an individual's training history. One of the drawbacks of a low-end system is that you may not be able to generate reports to show who has not taken a course or a report that can show you who is due for such courses as CPR recertification.

There are two other important items to consider in buying a training database: What kinds of hardware does the system need, and how many people will be using the system? Many small systems work on a basic PC (typically a single PC). They are not designed for use by multiple people from different areas; they allow one user at a time working at a solitary PC.

14. Is there a system that will meet the needs of a large education department?

If a basic training database is not going to meet your needs, it may be time to consider a training management system. These systems are much more sophisticated and, of course, cost much more money.

15. How much more do midlevel systems cost?

Midlevel systems are generally priced in the range of $10,000 and higher. There are also increased hardware costs. A midlevel system will run on your computer network from its own server. You need to include the cost of a server and any software needed to operate it. Another point to consider is that the costs of these systems are usually conditional and based on the number of users: the more users, the higher the price. It is also important to remember that the costs of these systems do not end with the purchase of software. In most cases, the system comes with a service contract, which may range from one-third to one-half of the original price and is paid on a yearly basis. At first you may think that you can live without this cost, but it is important to remember that the system is proprietary software; if it has an error (and it will), only the company that created it can correct the problem. It is actually much cheaper to pay the yearly bill than to have someone out of contract come in to fix the system ($2000 a day is not an uncommon fee level). Another important benefit to buying the service contract is upgrades. Most companies continuously improve their software. Each time that they make their system better, you will be given the improvements under the contract.

16. What kind of database do I need if I am dealing with thousands of employees?

For many institutions neither a basic nor a midlevel system is adequate because of the number of employees or the amount of information that needs to be included in the system. Imagine for a moment how many data are involved if you plan to store every course attended by every employee at your institution for a period of three years. (The three-year perspective would get you through only one JCAHO survey). It is easy to see that there will be millions of data points in the database in very short order. When databases become so large, it is often preferable to move beyond Access and into the realm of corporate databases.

Corporate databases usually do not belong to the education department alone. Corporate databases may be part of the institution's human resource or payroll system. They use multiple layers of software. The database itself may be Oracle, SQL, or DB. The positive aspect of this part of the system is that educators can give technical problems to the information systems department to worry about. These databases are often so big and so important to the company that a database manager is hired to make sure that they run correctly.

Since the database is taken care of, educators need to worry about the upper layer of software. Such systems are usually called the training record or management system. If you work with a system that is integrated with human resources or some other department, you are dealing with proprietary software that your institution has purchased as part of an overall package. Examples include PeopleSoft and Lawson HR software. The nice part about these systems is that the data related to the employees are put into the system by some other department (usually human resources), but you have access to the information. They are great time savers, but at this point some of the more advanced capabilities are limited.

17. Are even more advanced systems available?

Definitely. Recent advances in database and Internet technology have led to the development of highly sophisticated systems that actually manage the entire learning process. These systems are known as learning management systems (LMSs). The LMS is the next stage of development of education software.

18. What is a learning management system?

LMSs seem to have a different definition depending on the source. Some experts say that an LMS is used to provide web-based training through a portal type of system. Others explain how an LMS can track training records in a web-based format. Most define an LMS as a system to design, build, and operate web-based training for large numbers of people anywhere around the world. All of these definitions are true to some extent. LMSs are Internet-based systems that have the ability to provide, track, and report on training that takes place anywhere within a business.

Currently available LMSs were first designed for large global corporations such as Boeing or General Motors. Imagine for a moment that instead of being responsible for the training of 2000 health care workers at one hospital, you are responsible for 10,000 staff members stationed in 20 countries. You have just been given the assignment of providing training for a new product to every one of the 10,000 people. How would you do it? At this scale the LMS is an absolute necessity.

19. What functions of the LMS makes it different from a training database?

Training database systems have the ability to track training records according to the data that are entered into the system. The LMS goes far beyond this step. For most people in education, the LMS can bring order to the chaos that is created when educators use mixed forms of training. Lecture, video, CBT, WBT, and other forms of training create a tracking nightmare for educators. The LMS provides a single point from which all of these processes can be tracked. Training that is done as lecture or in some other noncomputer format is tracked by the LMS in the same way as in any of the systems already discussed. The data are collected and then manually entered into the system. When CBT and WBT are part of training, the LMS really shows its stuff. The LMS allows employees to launch these forms of training whenever and wherever they may be. It tracks the process through the program and can provide a test at the end of the program to assess what learning has taken place. The LMS stores all of its information in a large database system such as Oracle. The education department can generate reports about these data to see what is being done by employees and what value their training provides for the company.

Scheduling and registration for training are nightmares for any educator. Using an LMS, the process can be reduced to a few simple clicks. Examples of scheduling function in the LMS include room management, equipment scheduling, course scheduling, instructor scheduling, and even student scheduling. Student scheduling is particularly exciting for educators. Using CPR classes (the nightmare of every nursing staff educator) as an example, the process of scheduling in an LMS would go as follows. At the beginning of each year, the CPR classes would be set up in the system, and rooms would be reserved in the scheduling function. One month before the two-year anniversary of the CPR class, the LMS would send out an e-mail notice, reminding the employee of the impending need for CPR renewal. The employee would access the LMS and schedule him- or herself for a class. The educator does nothing in the system until the class is completed. The entire process of scheduling can be automated except for the initial set-up of the class. Some systems are so sophisticated that you can assign instructors to a class, and they automatically receive notification of dates and time as well as a list of what equipment they will need for the class.

The LMS is a convenience not only for the education department. Having an LMS puts the education process more effectively into the hands of the employee. Employees do not need to depend on the calendar to receive training. With the LMS and CBT/WBT training, employees can have real-time training when they need it. The comfortable thought is that this training can be done during downtime. The LMS goes beyond that. For example, an employee who must deal with a new piece of equipment can access the necessary training just as he or she is ready to begin using it. Think of how such training is currently provided: we bring everyone to a demonstration of the equipment and then send them back to their jobs for several weeks, after which they finally get to use the equipment. Do any of us actually remember what was done in the demonstration? If the demonstration is a CBT hooked to the LMS, it is available when needed for the employee—a true example of just-in-time training.

Another important aspect of the LMS is the ability to deploy training quickly and efficiently to staff wherever they may be located. Some changes affect everyone in the institution: hazardous material training, changes to hospital security, and changes in universal precautions. When these situations arose in the past, the staff would be forced to attend round-the-clock training sessions or some other house-wide training method. With the LMS in place, this type of training can be "pushed" to all staff. If the content can be created as a CBT, then everyone uses it through the LMS. An LMS can also deploy and track something as simple as an employee's reading of a policy or memo. You can even create a short competency test to ensure comprehension of key points. For example, you can place the restraint policy onto the LMS for employees to read, attach a competency test, and then track each employee's completion of the task. The LMS is a great way to train large numbers of people in a short period and still ensure that they understand the content.

20. Can the LMS be used to create CBT or WBT?

Yes and no. Some LMSs have authoring software, but it may be an additional cost. Many types of computerized training authoring programs are currently on the market. Products such as Toolbook II, Designers Edge, Course Builder, and Quest Net can make CBT/WBT programs that work with the LMS. The real question is whether you have the time and resources to produce this type of training. Many institutions that rely heavily on CBT/WBT have subdepartments specializing in the development of such courses. You could buy CBT/WBT training from other companies and have them connected to your LMS. Not all CBT/WBT programs, however, are compatible with all LMSs. Industry standards are under development, but they are only in their early stages. Make sure that you ask about compatibility before you buy CBT/WBT authoring software and the LMS.

In regard to creating CBT/WBT programs, some LMS companies discuss a learning content management system (LCMS). The LCMS is not an authoring tool; it is a way of creating training for the future. The best way to think of the LCMS is to take a course that you teach, chop it into small sections, and determine whether any of these sections can be used as part of another class. The LCMS does exactly this with CBT/WBT. Instead of building an entire program as a single unit, each part is broken into what is called an object. You then piece objects together to create the training program. The concept already is used in other industries, but only now is it making its way into health care. The LCMS is likely to be part of the future of staff education.

21. Where is the best place to purchase the CBT/WBT programs to run through the LMS?

The best way to deal with this problem is through the LMS vendor. If you do not have the resources to create CBT/WBT, consider buying an LMS that comes with training content as part of the package. Many of the Internet-based LMSs for health care come with hundreds of programs already connected to the system, such as yearly mandatory programs (e.g., fire, electrical system) and clinical programs for nursing and medicine. Some even include computer program training. By buying the programs as part of the package, you can save money and provide a greater range of training. The best part is that all of these programs are provided as training across the Internet.

22. Since the LMS is so efficient, should every hospital consider buying one?

The LMSs currently on the market have one great drawback—cost. The first question is always, "How much is it going to cost?" With an LMS, the initial numbers may be shocking. Most fully capable LMSs start at around $50,000 and can easily exceed $100,000. Yearly costs are in the same range because in most cases you buy LMS services from the vendor. Pricing is usually determined by multiplying the number of staff using the system times the number of programs to which they will have access during the year.

Of course, hidden costs also are involved. The LMS does not manage itself. Someone must administer the system on a regular basis. Information must be entered, and reports must be created. Maintaining the program is also an issue. Programs that you buy from the vendor must be customized to fit your policies. This is especially important with the JCAHO-related programs. If you are considering such a system, it is important to make these issues clear to senior administrators, who may think the LMS is a tool for replacing trainers.

23. How do I justify any of these systems?

Look to the benefits. First of all, there are the benefits to the education department. Such systems are designed to provide record keeping, record analysis, departmental cost analysis, and, in the case of the LMS, course management. Even the midlevel systems are designed to include cost information about every class entered into the system. If you are interested in tracking the costs of a class, these systems allow you to input the cost of materials and/or the cost of instructors. If you are more interested in who is teaching classes and when they teach, these systems can track class instructors. Instructors may be internal staff whom you want to track for credit or external instructors whom you track for costs. Some of the systems have class registration abilities. An issue always facing an instructor is who is coming to class. With a training management system, you can register people and generate a class roster before the class begins. The registration is also a great way of tracking who showed up for class and who did not.

An important benefit for the entire institution is the ability to create reports. Reports, of course, track events, class attendance, deficiencies, overdue certifications, and other variables. For the education department, the benefit is most clear when reports are needed for reviews such as JCAHO or OSHA. Consider what the cost would be for your hospital if a type I problem is noted because documentation of education is missing. The loss of prestige in the community alone can easily cost more than the price of a system.

The best way to justify these systems is by doing a cost analysis of the educational process. First, you need to analyze the cost of training in its present form. Break down the total into individual costs. It is crucial to know the per-person expenditures because the cost of the system is justified at this level. The yearly cost of $50,000 breaks down to $100.00 per person if you have 500 employees and $10.00 per person if you have 5000 employees. It is doubtful that any education department can provide training this cheaply on a consistent basis.

Unfortunately, nursing educators tend to think frugally. This tendency may be due to years of worry about how many washcloths were used today, but we need to lose such inhibitions. Other department managers have spent hundreds of thousands of dollars on projects to improve the corporate system, but educators have not. Educators needs to realize that this level of expense is not out of range. We must learn to do a cost-benefit analysis to justify the expense of a training management system.

24. How do I find the companies that provide the necessary software?

Training database applications are available from many companies. Listing names would be a futile process. By the time you read this chapter, the names may have changed. Thus, it is better to do an Internet search for the information. Try searching for information using keywords such as training or education management systems and learning management systems. Do not confine the search to health care because most of this information will be found under training and development. Another valuable source of information about these systems is the training and development journals. You need to think outside the box. Forget about health care, and look at the broad spectrum of training that is done in corporations.

25. What lies the future for the computer and the staff educator?

There will always be managers who see computers as a way to reduce the number of people or even eliminate jobs. For educators, computers are only tools for the enhancement of teaching. Computers cannot do the whole job. An educator needs to integrate what the computer teaches with the reality of the clinical environment. Computers also offer variety. We no longer need to do repetitive lectures on such issues as fire safety or proper hand washing. The computer can teach such subjects for us.

Where will we be in 5 or 10 years? At this point it seems as though the sky is the limit. The Internet continues to grow, and education is one of the biggest growth areas. The ability to get information on the Internet improves every day. In a few years, creating web-based training may be as easy as creating a lecture. With the expansion of the Internet, the world continues to shrink. Internet-based LMSs are going to be a large part of growth in the Internet world. As LMSs improve, costs will decrease, and applicability will expand. The LMS will allow expansion of education in ways that we have yet to conceive.

In addition, in the future you may be collaborating with staff educators across the country to provide high-quality programs. Every hospital may be able to use national and even international experts to provide specialty training. The student population will change along with the technology. The teenagers of today are the clinical staff of the future. Having been raised on Nintendo and PlayStation, will they really be willing to sit for hours listening to a lecture? We need to adapt to their wants and needs. In 5 or 10 years, we may be able to simulate real patient environments in a virtual hospital. Think of what it would be like to have an employee go through ACLS as a virtual simulation. Think of how much easier and less stressful it would be to assess competency with a new procedure in a virtual hospital than at a patient's bedside. The future holds many new and exciting tools for the staff educator.

BIBLIOGRAPHY

1. Brandon-Hall Staff: E-Learning Guidebook: Six Steps to Implementing E-Learning. Available at www.brandonhall.com/public/pdfs/sixstepguidebook.pdf.
2. Commission on Technology and Adult Learning: A Vision of E-Learning Workforce for America. Available at www.astd.org/virtual_community/public_policy/jh_ver.pdf.
3. Hartnett J: Why Johnny can't read wbt: How to write for the web. Inside Technol Train 4:60–65, 2000.
4. Masie E: The Computer Training Handbook: Strategies for Helping People to Learn Technology. Minneapolis, MN, Lakewood Books, 1998.
5. Shepherd C: A Day in the Life of a Leaning Management System. TACTIX: Training and Communications Technology in Context. Available at www.fastrak-consulting.co.uk/tactix/features/lms/lms.htm
6. Singh H: New technologies for new learning approaches. E-learning 2(2):36–38, 53, 2001.
7. Wolford R, Hughes L: Using the hospital intranet to meet competency standards for nurses. J Nurs Staff Devel 17:182–189, 2001.

17. EVALUATION

Rebecca Wilson, MSN, RN, C, *Cynthia Crockett*, MSN, RN,
and Belinda Curtis, BSN, RN, BC

1. Define evaluation.

Although the term *evaluation* has many different meanings, common threads generally include measurement and judgment components. Evaluation also may refer to the appraisal of a course or to the level of achievement of individual participants in terms of learning objectives. Evaluation is the process by which a judgment is made about the relative value of something. Evaluation should be built into all educational services.

2. Why is evaluation essential in educational services?

Evaluation is an important aspect of staff development services. It is invaluable in determining the quality of education. Staff development educators recognize many reasons for evaluating. The greatest effect of staff development evaluations lies in the ability to demonstrate the transference of learning to the bedside. Other primary reasons for evaluating are (1) to measure the achievement of learning outcomes, (2) to justify the existence of the organizational learning function, (3) to decide whether to continue or discontinue specific learning opportunities, and (4) to gain information about how to improve future learning opportunities. Secondary reasons for evaluating include meeting accreditation/approval requirements, accounting for funds, making administrative decisions, and assisting in program development.

3. What framework is available to help me in planning an evaluation?

Think about evaluation as a process with five possible levels:

Level 1 evaluation is concerned with participant satisfaction with the educational activity.

Level 2 measures the degree of learning.

Level 3 evaluates outcomes or transference of learning to the work area.

Level 4 evaluates the effect of the program on the organization as a whole.

Level 5 addresses return on investment (ROI).

It is not necessary to evaluate every educational offering at all levels. It is important, however, to include all of the supportive levels up to the highest level that you choose. For example, you may design an evaluation that measures outcomes but does not include an evaluation of learning. If the outcome evaluation shows little improvement, a major question remains unanswered: is the lack of improvement due to failure of participants to learn or to difficulty in the transfer of learning?

Levels of Evaluation for the Implementation of a New Web-based EKG Course

LEVEL	FOCUS	EXAMPLE
1	Participant satisfaction	Participants complete an evaluation form at the completion of the course and answer questions such as the following: • How satisfied are you with this new type of course? • Were you able to meet the objectives of the course? • Did you encounter any technical difficulty? • Would you recommend this web-based course to others? • What would have improved it?
2	Knowledge: has learning occurred?	Participants take a test when they compete the web-based course and must receive an 80% or better.
3	Transference of learning: Can the participant perform in his/her clinical area?	Participants are expected to read EKGs in their clinical area with accuracy. Instructors/preceptors check EKG analysis of participants for accuracy.

Continued on following page

Levels of Evaluation for the Implementation of a New Web-based EKG Course (Continued)

LEVEL	FOCUS	EXAMPLE
4	Impact: What is the effect of this program on the organization as a whole?	Analysis of the course to determine organizational effect of of the new website-based EKG course: • More flexibility for staff, especially staff who are unable to attend classes during the day; increased opportunities for nurses to gain employment on telemetry unit • Decreased cost: web-based course took ___ the time of the instructor-led course, saving staff salaries, replacement staff salaries, and instructor salaries • Improved quality of care
5	Return on investment (ROI)	ROI is calculated (see question 26)

4. How do I know that the educational activity I am planning will work?

Testing your materials or offerings for effectiveness is known as formative evaluation, which usually is done near the end of the development phase. The educator(s) closely involved in the design and development of the activity typically carry out this evaluation. The first phase entails review of the materials by a content expert for completeness and accuracy. The next phase is to form a pilot group that is representative of the target audience (also known as a beta test). The pilot group for a self-directed learning package should consist of at least three evaluators, preferably one who is a novice, one who is an average performer, and one who is a high performer in the topic or skill to be covered. When evaluating a presentation, you want to gather information about participant satisfaction and achievement of the learning objectives. For a self-directed learning package, obtain information about clarity of the directions and materials, satisfaction with the package itself, achievement of the learning objectives, and time required for completion. Modifications then can be made before wider distribution of the learning activity.

5. What is involved in level 1 evaluation?

The most common approach is to ask participants to complete an evaluation form immediately after an educational activity to capture their reactions. The American Nurses' Credentialing Center Commission on Accreditation (ANCC-COA) recommends at a minimum collecting data about the following aspects:

1. Relationship of objectives to the overall purpose/goals of the activity
2. Learner achievement of each objective
3. Expertise of each individual presenter
4. Appropriateness of teaching strategies
5. Appropriateness of physical facilities

Various forms have been developed to collect this information. Such forms often contain a mixture of closed-ended Likert-type questions and open-ended questions. Closed-ended questions can be measured on a scale from low to high satisfaction. An example of an open-ended question is, "Which part of the activity was most or least useful to you?" The key to using this method of evaluation is to attain as close to a 100% completion rate as possible. One strategy for achieving this goal is to build evaluation time into the schedule.

6. Discuss the benefit of evaluating participant satisfaction.

Evaluation of participant satisfaction provides educators with information that can be used for a variety of purposes. Feedback and suggestions provided by participants can be used to improve future offerings. Participant ratings also may be used as part of the educators' overall performance evaluation. For participants, providing feedback confirms that their input is valuable to the education staff. In addition, participants who are not satisfied with the offering are less likely to be motivated to learn and/or return to an educational program. Managers also use this information as a basis for supporting participation in future educational offerings. Sample participant evaluation forms are found in Appendices A and B.

7. Describe level 2 evaluation.

Measurement of learning involves determining one or more of the following:

- What knowledge was gained (cognitive domain)
- What skills were developed or improved (psychomotor domain)
- What attitudes were changed (affective domain)

Learning is measured at the conclusion of the educational activity.

8. What level 2 evaluation methods are appropriate for adult learners?

Pretest and posttest. This method is commonly used to measure gains in knowledge or the cognitive domain. Although many adults do not like to take tests, they provide a measure of learning that can be used for evaluation purposes. Changing the title from "test" to "evaluation of learning" or "learning assessment" may be perceived as less threatening to the learner. Using a pretest/posttest method helps to determine the level of knowledge that participants possessed before the educational activity and changes related to their participation. A pretest is not necessary if you believe that the participants do not possess a base knowledge before the course (e.g., introducing a new piece of equipment). Specific data points can be analyzed to provide information that will guide the educator to alter the content or teaching strategies to improve learner outcomes.

Question-and-answer session. With an interactive lecture, the educator can gauge the effectiveness of teaching by the types of questions posed by the learners. A skilled educator can evaluate learner knowledge level, and continuously modify the curriculum based on the types of questions asked by the audience. By keeping the question-and-answer session focused on the audience and course objectives, the educator can clarify topics for the audience and more likely achieve the stated objectives.

Open-ended questions. A simple method to gain general information about degree of learning is to ask open-ended questions related to what the participant has learned and how the participant will use this information. This approach provides data about what participants found to be important and helps the participants to begin thinking about how they can use the information in their work area.

Observation. The learner's acquisition of psychomotor skills is often measured by use of observation or return demonstration. Development of a skills checklist assists the educator with consistency in evaluation. These checklists include all of the critical elements and the order in which they are to be performed. An example is the checklist of skills used during a basic life support course.

Survey. Attitudes can be measured with a survey administered before and after an educational activity. The survey targets the attitudes that participants should possess after attending the program. A comparison of the pre- and postsurvey results indicates what changes, if any, occurred as a result of the activity. For example, if a participant objective states that learners will recognize the importance of assessing a patient's cultural background as it relates to their care, a survey question would ask participants to state the value of performing such an assessment.

9. What else should I keep in mind when doing a level 2 evaluation?

The evaluation process should measure whether learning objectives were attained and then make a decision or judgment about the level of attainment (e.g., how well participants met the objectives: A, B, C, D, F; pass/fail).

A key point in evaluating learning is to make sure to align your evaluation with your learning objectives. It is frustrating for participants to be asked about information that was not part of the activity. Ask "So what?" before adding a question to a test. Methods of evaluation also must be congruent. For example, if the learning objectives lie within the cognitive domain (e.g., describe, discuss, analyze), the evaluation should not include a skill checklist (e.g., demonstrate, perform). Creating valid measures of learning is among the most difficult challenges facing staff development educators.

10. How do I know whether a test is valid (i.e., it measures what I intend to measure)?

There are many aspects to determining the validity of a test. Two nonstatistical measures are face-validity and content-validity. Subject experts judge the test in terms of accuracy and comprehensiveness to determine face validity. Content-related validity refers to how the test aligns with the objectives and cognitive level required. It is often the most important type of validity for staff development. Standardized tests often have statistical measures of validity, which are available from the publisher. You may choose to purchase standardized tests, such as those published by the National League for Nursing. The most critical factor in testing is to make sure that the test fits your institution's needs in terms of competency. It is advisable to pilot the test on a small group to determine its suitability.

11. What about reliability?

Tests need to be reliable as well as valid. Reliability describes whether a test or other evaluation method measures consistently. Reliability is important because it tells you basically whether your test scores are free of error caused by the test itself. Standardized tests provide reliability statistics. Your research department can help you determine the reliability of tests that you develop.

12. How do I measure retention of information?

A follow-up posttest is needed. A posttest can be conducted immediately after the program and 1 month after the program to measure knowledge retention.

13. How do I measure level 3 outcomes?

Level 3 evaluations measure changes in the learner's behavior that are evident in the work environment. The difficulty in measuring outcomes lies in the number of variables that influence transferral of knowledge to everyday practice. For behavioral change, the learner needs the knowledge and skills to perform and a work environment that supports the change. In an effort to control for these variables, methods used for outcome measurement are similar to those used in research.

Level 3 evaluation takes place in the work setting and is not measured until the participant has the opportunity to use the new behavior. Occasionally, the opportunity arises soon after the participants return to the clinical area. For example, a nurse may be asked to manage the care of a dying patient soon after returning from a course about the emotional care of dying patients. You may observe the implementation of key strategies emphasized in the educational offering. For programs that are extensive in nature, changes manifest more slowly. These differences influence the timing of the evaluation, which may not be appropriate until 3–6 months after the educational activity. The amount and type of data collected depend on the purpose and intended audience of the evaluation.

Data collection includes surveys and interviews from participants (self-report), managers, peers, or others who have an opportunity to observe participant behavior. Kirkpatrick[7] suggests two simple open-ended questions: "Are you doing anything different since you attended the educational program?" and "Why or why not?" Other methods for determining outcomes include direct observation of participant behavior, changes in documentation, or changes in processes or policies. It is beneficial to use more than one method of data collection to support your analysis.

14. What is a level 4 evaluation?

Impact evaluation focuses on organizational results derived from education. This level of evaluation is more global and looks for improvements in areas such as quality of patient care, number of safety or incident reports, turnover, and cost-effectiveness. For example, if quality data revealed a high level of central line infections, educational sessions about central line maintenance and care may be offered. If data collected after the activity show a decrease in line infections and shortened length of stay, the educational sessions are shown to affect quality and cost-effectiveness of care. These data, supported by evaluation of learning and outcomes, provide evidence that educational activities result in improvement.

15. Should I evaluate outcomes and impact for every educational activity?

It is not feasible or necessary to measure outcomes and impact for every activity. The decision is based on the relative costs and benefits of the evaluation. Evaluating outcomes of educational activities is costly in terms of staff time or consultant fees if the evaluation is extensive or complex. Data collection is relatively inexpensive, because the necessary data are often available within the organization.

In general, the importance of performing an outcome or impact evaluation increases directly with the expense and scope of the proposed program. Factors to consider in determining the advisability of level 3 evaluation include program cost, number of times the program is to be offered, number of staff participating, and potential results of the evaluation (e.g., decisions about continuing the program). These factors are balanced against the cost in staff time and tool development or acquisition. In general, impact evaluation is recommended for programs that are high volume, high risk, high cost, or problem-prone.

16. When do I start planning the evaluation of a new offering or program?

One key to successful evaluation is to develop the evaluation plan during the initial planning stages. Planning includes defining the target audience and determining the scope, goal, and objectives of the activity. These factors provide the information needed to decide the level of evaluation. Design your evaluation to address the goals and objectives of the offering. For example, if one objective states that the participant will be able to demonstrate a particular skill, plan to evaluate evidence of learning with tools such as a skills checklist, case study, or role-play.

17. Explain summative evaluation. How does it relate to staff development?

The process of evaluating the overall effectiveness and fit of an educational activity with organizational goals is termed summative evaluation. The main goal of summative evaluation is to provide information to people responsible for deciding to continue or discontinue the offering or program. Summative evaluation is performed from the management perspective. To preserve objectivity, the evaluators should be persons who are not closely associated with development and implementation of the program.

Summative evaluation contains elements of outcome and impact evaluation. Data are collected to determine whether participants are able to transfer their learning and whether the change in behavior has a positive effect on the organization as a whole. In addition, issues such as implementation, usability, and cost-effectiveness are analyzed to support the decision.

For example, a hospital may have offered classes on cultural assessment every month for the past year. A summative evaluation examines the quality of cultural assessment, and patient satisfaction surveys indicate whether patients perceived staff interest in their individual needs.

18. How do I know if an offering or program is worth continuing?

Improvement in evaluation measures supports continuance of the class. Lack of change or a decrease in performance supports discontinuance of the current class and a search for alternative methods to address the need.

19. What about evaluating ongoing offerings or programs?

Ongoing programs, such as orientation or continuing education, need to be evaluated. There are no overall standards for how often an ongoing offering or program should be evaluated. Minimal standards are set by accrediting or regulatory agencies such as the ANCC-COA if your program is accredited. Participant evaluation of the program (level 1) is required (see question 5)

The evaluation process can be initiated when a program is found to be problem-prone or its cost-effectiveness is questioned. Changes in the external environment, such as new regulations or research, also prompt a need to evaluate current practice. Finally, changes in the internal environment (e.g., new equipment and procedures, a new organizational vision and mission) are also catalysts for evaluation.

20. What are the steps in performing a large program evaluation?

Puetz[8] identified six steps in planning a large program evaluation. An example may be evaluating the nursing orientation program. The key is to form a team of stakeholders that can support the planning.

1. **Identify the relevant stakeholders.** It is important to include representatives from areas that are affected by the program. This group includes representative administrators, educators, and program participants. An evaluation consultant (an external expert in evaluation methods and tools) also may be included, depending on the scope of the project and the expertise within the organization.

2. **Arrange preliminary meetings.** The purpose of these meetings is to gather information about the purpose, audience, resource requirements, and timeline for completing the evaluation. Data collected from these meetings are used in subsequent steps.

3. **Decide whether to evaluate.** Once the data have been collected about the benefits and costs of evaluation, the decision is made whether or not to proceed. It is advisable to proceed only if the benefits of evaluation outweigh the costs.

4. **Examine the literature.** Searching the literature for similar evaluation projects can save valuable time by reducing the need to reinvent a strategy. The literature can suggest appropriate designs, useful instruments for collecting data, and outcomes of similar evaluations.

5. **Determine the methods**. Once you have reviewed the literature, it is time to determine the methods by which the evaluation will be completed. This phase entails designing the overall plan and approach, identifying sources of data, selecting or developing data collection tools, and determining data collection methods.

6. **Present the proposal.** This is the final step before implementation. Often a written proposal is shared with relevant groups within an organization. The report should include sufficient detail for reviewers to understand the process.

21. What are the possible evaluation methods?

Various methods can be used in conducting an evaluation. It is important not to collect more data than can be used. It can be extremely frustrating and overwhelming to sift through countless papers in an attempt to derive the meaning of it all. For this reason, selecting a data collection method is an important component to consider early in the process. There are two basic methods of data analysis: quantitative (statistical analysis) and qualitative (analysis of patterns or themes).

22. How do quantitative and qualitative methods differ?

Quantitative methods define the relationships between variables or describe variables. Results are reported in terms of numbers and statistical significance. Tools frequently used to obtain quantitative data include questionnaires and surveys consisting of closed-ended questions and multiple choice testing to measure learning.

Qualitative methods gather subjective data based on participant experiences and opinions. The purpose of qualitative methods is to observe the occurrence of variables in a natural setting. The qualitative approach uses pattern identification or theme analysis. Data collection occurs in the practice setting using tools such as interviews and observation.

23. What about continuous quality improvement methods?

Numerous continuous quality improvement methods are available; all are based on the principles of baseline data collection, identification of causes, and development and implementation of new processes, followed by data collection to measure improvement against goals set. The educator measures change in processes that reflect the effectiveness of the learning. Become familiar with the method used by your hospital or health system for continuous quality improvement.

24. How do I demonstrate the financial value of education?

Current methods for demonstrating the dollar value of education to the organization include cost-effectiveness analysis, cost-benefit analysis, and return on investment. Common to all of these methods is calculating the cost of providing the education and comparing it with the impact on the organization.

Program Costs

CATEGORIES OF COST	EXAMPLES
Learner	Salary and benefits
Instructor	Salary and benefits for development, implementation, and evaluation of the program Travel, food, lodging
Support personnel	Salaries and benefits
Material resources	Promotional materials Supplies Printing and duplication services Facility costs

Cost-effectiveness analysis measures the efficacy of a program in achieving outcomes in relation to what it costs. Usually cost-effectiveness is expressed as cost per unit of outcomes achieved. In comparison, cost-benefit analysis measures the efficacy of a program expressed as the relation between costs and outcomes, usually in monetary terms. Return on investment is similar to a cost-benefit analysis, but the formula differs slightly and is expressed as percent returned.

25. How do I perform a cost-effectiveness analysis?

In performing a cost-effectiveness analysis, total program costs are identified and calculated. The next step is to divide the total cost by the number of participants to derive the cost per participant. Effectiveness ratings are based on the level of evaluation that will be used to assess the outcomes of the educational activity.

Cost-effectiveness Analysis Worksheet

Costs

Learner salaries __________
Instructor salary __________
Development time/salary __________
Materials __________
Facilities __________
Evaluation/assessment of learning __________
Cost per participant hour (total costs/number of participants) __________
Calculate or estimate average learner salary __________
Convert to cost value such as __________

1 = average learner salary + $20
2 = average learner salary + $15
3 = average learner salary + $10
2 = average learner salary + $5
1 = average learner salary + $1

Effectiveness

Select an effectiveness value based on actual evaluation method and data such as: __________

1 = evidence that participants were present in the room
2 = evidence that participants learned in class (written or performance tests, direct observation, expressed change in attitude)
3 = evidence that majority of participants transferred learning to work setting as noted through direct observation
4 = evidence that majority of participants transferred learning to work setting noted by quality monitoring activity
5 = evidence that majority of participants transferred learning to work setting noted through data collected by unobtrusive evaluation measures

Continued on following page

Cost-effectiveness Analysis Worksheet (Continued)

Compare cost to effective value ________
1:1 = poor use of scarce resources, no outcomes
3:3 = good use of scarce resources, classroom outcomes
5:5 = ask for a raise (you can reach this level with planning)

Address your findings in your continuous improvement plans and reports.

Source: Karen Kelly-Thomas, 1997, used with permission. Modified from formula developed by Dorothy del Bueno, 1980.

26. How do I determine cost-benefit or return on investment (level 5 evaluation)?

Cost-benefit analysis and ROI start with total program costs. The next step is to collect data about the outcomes and impact on the organization. From these data, isolate effects that are attributable to the educational offering. Designing an evaluation that determines outcomes and requests participants, managers, and administration to estimate impact on the organization will assist in isolating these effects. Hard data, such as increased productivity or decreased length of stay, can be translated into monetary terms. Quantifying soft data, such as patient satisfaction, is a highly subjective process that requires the evaluators to estimate their financial impact. The few benefits that cannot be translated into monetary terms are noted as "intangible" benefits in the analysis. This method works best when most of the outcomes are more directly related to financial impact, such as decreased patient length of stay or increased productivity.

For cost-benefit analysis, the final result is expressed as a ratio of:

$$\frac{\text{Program benefits}}{\text{Total program costs}}$$

For ROI, the formula uses net program benefits (program benefits – program costs) and is expressed as a percentage of return on investment:

$$\frac{\text{Net program benefit}}{\text{Program costs}} \times 100$$

For example, the total cost (including development, instructor time, learner time, supplies, and evaluation) of a program designed to reduce central line infections is $4,000. The outcome of the program is an 80% reduction in line infections. This reduction leads to savings in laboratory work, line replacement, additional antibiotic therapy, and shortened length of stay. These benefits, expressed in monetary terms, are estimated at $10,000 per year. The cost-benefit formula is as follows:

$$\frac{\$10{,}000}{\$4{,}000} = \$2.5 \text{ in benefit for every dollar spent on the program}$$

The ROI formula is as follows:

$$\frac{\$10{,}000 - \$4{,}000}{\$4{,}000} \times 100 = 150\% \text{ ROI}$$

Evaluating cost-benefit and ROI is not feasible for every educational activity. Isolating the effects of training and quantifying soft data are definite challenges in evaluating the financial rewards of education.

27. How do I share evaluation data with the staff?

Many staff development educators use evaluation summaries to provide feedback to staff about a program, workshop, or course that they attended. Summaries can be posted in the staff bathrooms and on bulletin boards in the nursing units and/or electronically mailed to participants. If the results of the evaluation will lead to changes in the course before it is offered again, such information should be communicated to prior participants. This approach gives staff the reassurance that their opinions count and that they can help initiate change. It can also encourage the future success of courses if staff trust and value the educational process.

Specific evaluation data should be shared with individual instructors. Be cautious to protect the confidentiality and self-esteem of instructors within a group course if one of the instructors received negative comments.

28. What do I need to consider when sharing evaluation results with management and administration?

Compile the data and select a reporting format based on the preferences of the administrators and managers who comprise your target audience and the medium for presentation. One common format is the executive summary, a short document (1–2 pages) that presents only key points supplemented with appropriate data. Information is emphasized by the use of bullet points. Take the preparation of this document seriously, because it offers an opportunity to educate others about the program. Quantitative data are more easily understood in the form of a chart or graph. Information represented in this portion of the report may include ROI or cost-benefit ratio. Qualitative data are reported in narrative or short-sentence format. The report also should include the actual number of staff who participated in the educational activity and percentages of participants who participated in the evaluation (e.g., 100% of participants completed the reaction and learning evaluation; 80% returned a post-class survey). This information is useful in determining staff participation or compliance in the case of mandatory attendance. Finally, it is important to consider what factors promoted or limited the success of the program. Will any of the lessons learned improve your program in the future?

BIBLIOGRAPHY

1. Alspach JG: The Educational Process in Nursing Staff Development. St. Louis, Mosby, 1995.
2. Brunt BA: Continuing education evaluation of behavior change. J Nurs Staff Devel 16:49–54, 2000.
3. Case B: Competence development, critical thinking, clinical judgment, and technical ability. In Kelly-Thomas KJ (ed): Clinical and Nursing Staff Development: Current Competence, Future Focus, 2nd ed. Philadelphia, J. B. Lippincott, 1998, pp 241–281.
4. Dick W, Carey L, Carey JO: The Systematic Design of Instruction, 5th ed. New York, Addison-Wesley , 2001.
5. Homes SA: Getting started. J Nurs Staff Devel 6:204–207, 1990.
6. Jeska SB, Fischer KJ: Performance Improvement in Staff Development: The Next Evolution. Pensacola, FL, National Nursing Staff Development Organization, 1996.
7. Kelly-Thomas KJ (ed): Clinical and Nursing Staff Development: Current Competence, Future Focus, 2nd ed. Philadelphia, J.B.Lippincott, 1998, p 360.
8. Kirkpatrick DL: Evaluating Training Programs: The Four Levels. San Francisco, Berrett-Koehler, 1994.
9. Puetz BE: Evaluation in Nursing Staff Development: Methods and Models. Gaithersburg, MD, Aspen, 1985.
10. Sullivan H, Higgins N: Teaching for Competence. New York, Teacher's College Press, 1983.

Appendix A: Course Evaluation Form

SAMPLE EVALUATION FORM

COURSE NAME:

DATE :

DIRECTIONS: On a scale from 1 to 5, with 5 being the highest, rate the following by placing a mark in the box under the number that applies.

EVALUATION OF SPEAKER:

Speaker	Expertise of Presenter / Faculty					Effectiveness of Teaching Method				
	5	4	3	2	1	5	4	3	2	1

		5	4	3	2	1
1.	Please rate the extent to which the objectives of this course were related to the overall goal. <Insert Goal Here>					
2.	Please rate the extent to which you were able to achieve each objective.					
a.						
b.						
c.						
d.						
e.						
3.	Please rate the extent to which your personal objectives were met.					
4.	How would you rate the appropriateness of the physical facilities, including room, location, etc.?					

5. **What part of the program was most helpful?**

6. **Any suggestions for improvements?**

7. **Comments:**

From the Mayo Clinic, Phoenix, AZ, with permission.

Appendix B: Allied Health Orientation Feedback

1) How would you evaluate the orientation program overall?

___ Excellent ___ Very Good ___ Good ___ Fair ___ Poor

2) From orientation, what do you think < Institution Name> stands for?

____

3) From orientation, what do you think is expected of you as an employee?

____

4) Describe how to gain access to policies.

____

5) Please rate the effectiveness of the presentations on a scale of 1-5, with 1 being not effective, 5 being very effective. Mark N/A if you did not attend a particular class.

Topic	5	4	3	2	1

Comments:

Thank you for sharing your feedback with us

From the Mayo Clinic, Phoenix, AZ, with permission.

IV. *The Nuts and Bolts of Common Nursing Staff Development Programs*

18. ORIENTATION

Roxanne Amerson, MSN, RN, BC

1. Standards of the Joint Commission for Accrediation of Healthcare Organizations (JCAHO) refer to competency-based orientation (CBO). What is meant by CBO?

A competency-based education program focuses on the learner's ability to perform a task rather than simple possession of the knowledge required to perform the task. An agency identifies specific competencies that a person must demonstrate to be considered competent to deliver client care as well as the specific competency and the minimal level at which the task must be demonstrated. A CBO program is based on andragogy, which involves adult learning principles with an outcome-based plan of evaluation.

2. Explain the three essential components of a CBO program.

The three essential components of a CBO program are competency statements, critical behaviors, and learning options. The competency statements are the performance outcomes that an employee is expected to demonstrate. The critical behaviors are the specific actions that must be completed to meet the competency statements. For example, a critical behavior for the dressing change of a central line is maintenance of sterile technique. Finally, the program identifies a variety of learning options to assist the employee to perform the identified behaviors.

3. What are the advantages of a CBO program?

The major advantage of the CBO program is that it decreases the time spent on orientation of new staff. In addition, staff are expected to have a uniform knowledge base at the end of the program and to possess the skills required to provide safe, effective client care. The designated competency statements and critical behaviors provide validation of the staff member's level of skill. This type of program clearly identifies for the preceptor the expectations that should be demonstrated by the new staff member during the clinical experience. New staff are able to recognize their own strengths and weaknesses based on their performance of the critical behaviors necessary for completion of the competency.

4. Discuss the barriers to implementing an effective orientation program.

One major barrier to implementation of an orientation program is the inconsistency or lack of adequate preceptor education about the CBO program. Preceptors must have a clear understanding of the CBO process and the expectations of the overall program. Secondly, it is important that implementation of the program be standardized throughout the institution. Competencies and competency statements may vary based on the unit and the type of health care delivery, but all units within the institution should be following the same format for actual completion of the competency validation. The majority of the required competencies should focus on high-risk, high-volume, or high-risk, low-volume procedures. Competencies that focus on low-volume, low-risk procedures usually do not benefit the institution or the individual employee.

5. What are the critical elements that need to be covered in an orientation program?

Orientation needs vary, depending on the institution and the delivery of care specific to that institution. The critical elements of an orientation program generally involve the mandatory issues required by regulating agencies (e.g., JCAHO, Occupational Safety and Health Administration [OSHA]); payroll compensation and benefits; policies and procedures specific to the institution; and assessment of competency for role-specific duties, documentation, and equipment.

6. How do I differentiate between institutional-wide orientation and departmental orientation?

Institutional-wide orientation (sometimes called hospital orientation) involves the introduction to information that is required of every employee, regardless of job title or position. This type of orientation generally consists of mandatory issues (e.g., fire and safety, infection control, customer relations), payroll compensation, and benefits. Departmental orientation involves the policies, procedures, and equipment that are more specific to the unique area of patient care delivery within the institution. The departmental orientation also introduces the employee to a job-specific orientation that involves the employee's specific duties.

7. How does the employee's level of experience affect orientation?

Most institutions currently use some form of CBO, which theoretically allows the employee to progress more quickly through the orientation process based on level of experience. Experienced nurses should be expected to progress in a shorter period than new graduate nurses. Many institutions have developed longer, more in-depth programs for new graduate nurses. CBO focuses on the premise that the nurse will demonstrate his or her current knowledge level and be required to attend only educational sessions that address areas of patient care in which the nurse cannot demonstrate a predetermined level of minimal competency. Thus, an experienced nurse is expected to demonstrate competency in most routine nursing procedures without instruction in a short period.

8. Is there an average length of time for orientation?

Orientation length is highly variable. It depends on multiple factors, such as the structure and integration of institution-wide orientation with department orientation, the method of instruction for orientation issues, the level and acuity of patient care of the select setting, and budgetary constraints, to name a few. Most facilities allow 3–5 days of classroom instruction followed by 2–6 weeks of unit-specific training with an assigned preceptor. A new graduate nurse orientation program may last as long as 12 weeks. Internships for new graduates in specialty areas may last from 6 months to 1 year.

9. What type of documentation must be maintained in relation to orientation programs?

Each planned program should include a course outline with specific objectives, content to be covered, teaching strategies, and allotted time for completion. When competency validation is required, the educator should maintain records that clearly document the successful performance by the learner of the specified competencies. The documentation should be specific, objective, observable, and consistently applied to all learners. Performance criteria for competency should identify critical behaviors that establish a minimal performance level that is acceptable to demonstrate competency. Course outlines should be maintained within the education department, but documentation of competency validation usually is maintained by the employee's direct supervisor or within the human resources department. Competency validation should take place before the delivery of care to clients. Sample forms for documentation of CBO for a maternity nurse are found in Appendix A.

10. How is the orientation of a new graduate different from the normal orientation for an experienced nurse?

Although many areas overlap (e.g., introduction to the hospital policies for technical procedures or medication administration), it is important to focus on areas that are new to the graduate nurse. Graduate nurses frequently are still at the novice or advanced beginner stage of evaluating the client's response to treatment, clinical problem-solving, and prioritizing client care. The inexperienced nurse may benefit from assistance in planning and evaluating his or her professional development and teamwork behaviors. Initially biweekly evaluation may prove to be quite helpful in supporting the nurse in his or her new role. The frequency of the evaluations provides encouragement for positive behaviors and helps to correct deficiencies early in the orientation program.

11. How important is socialization during orientation? Does it have an effect on retention?

During orientation, new employees learn the values, expected behaviors, and essential knowledge that is required to perform their role within the institution. This learned behavior occurs through the process of socialization. Role transition is the process that a person experiences as he or she changes from a previous set of expectations to the expectations of the new employer. Successful role transition requires assimilation of the values of the new role and setting. Early experiences during orientation have a significant effect on the person's long-term performance. Inconsistencies in the values and behaviors demonstrated during orientation increase the probability of dissatisfaction in the role, anxiety, and poor performance. Based on these negative consequences, the likelihood of becoming frustrated and overwhelmed with new duties greatly increases the risk that the person will not remain at the institution. One institution noted that almost 90% of new graduate nurses were retained 1 year after the revision of the orientation program to provide a more comprehensive 12-week fellowship component.

12. Some staff members work within the institution for a number of years in one role and then complete a higher level of education. What type of orientation do they need for their new role?

In most cases, the employee does not need to attend the institution-wide orientation. He or she has worked with the institution and probably is quite familiar with the mandatory education that is provided on an annual basis. The person may need to attend specific mandatory classes if the information given previously was geared specifically for a particular level of care provider (e.g., infection control specific to the duties of a certified nursing assistant). The employee needs to attend any educational sessions that address duties that are unique to the new role.

13. What other orientation issues are involved for nurses recruited from foreign countries?

The orientation of international nurses involves involves numerous issues. Such nurses are adjusting not only to your facility but also to a new culture and a new country. Common problems include language (medical jargon as well as basic English), interpersonal communication differences, and differences in nursing education. International nurses may be deficient in certain content areas of information, study, and learning skills. An excellent resource is Alspach's *The Educational Process in Nursing Staff Development*, which lays out the important issues and provides excellent suggestions for supporting international nurses.

14. The education department is expected to providesorientation for both direct care staff and ancillary staff. What kind of variation can be expected in orientation length for the different groups?

Once mandated education has been completed, the groups should be separated and oriented in a manner that addresses unique aspects of their different roles. To devise an educational plan that makes efficient use of the educator and the new employees' time, it is important to compare duties and responsibilities of the different groups. The educational plan should take into account the common areas of patient care and then allow division into separate groups as duties become more specific (see sample plan below). A well-planned education curriculum prevents redundancy in teaching common areas of content by combining different disciplines into a larger group. The combination of groups with similar duties makes efficient use of the educator and employee orientation time.

DAY 1	DAY 2	DAY 3
Welcome	Cultural diversity	IV fluids and central lines
Fire and safety	Communication techniques	Blood product administration
Customer relations	Isolation cart procedures	Organ procurement procedures
Patients' Bill of Rights	Transfer technique	Oxygen therapy
Advance directives	Ethical dilemmas	Medication administration
Back safety	CPR certification	Nutritional support
Infection control	Restraints	Crash cart procedures

Day 1: All employees, including direct care staff and ancillary staff.

Day 2: Direct care staff (nurses, nursing assistants, transport staff, unit secretaries, housekeeping, therapists, therapy assistants) in the morning. After completion of communication techniques, unit secretaries and housekeeping staff return to department for unit-specific training.

Day 3: Only nurses remain for educational sessions. Employees in all other disciplines return to their department for unit-specific training.

15. What issues need to be considered in planning an orientation program for unlicensed assistive personnel (UAPs)?

UAPs most commonly consist of certified nursing assistants (CNAs), unit secretaries, orderlies, and telemetry monitor technicians. One of the most critical aspects in planning an educational program for UAPs is literacy level. Frequently the workforce available for these positions has low or minimal literacy skills. Although a high school diploma may be required for the position, it does not guarantee adequate reading or math abilities. Standardized testing early in the orientation or before employment can identify potential problems early and help the educator to provide adequate training methods and materials that accommodate a lower literacy level when necessary. Some institutions provide programs that assist employees with literacy deficits to improve their skills during their employment at the institution. The expected benefits of such programs include increased self-esteem, job loyalty, job performance, and improved morale.

Another significant concern with UAPs is lack of understanding of the rationale for planned interventions. Many UAPs have been taught how to perform a designated skill with little or no background knowledge of why the skill is performed or how it may affect the outcome of care for a specific client. For example, in some institutions, CNAs are taught to perform urinary catheterization for selected clients. The basic training of a CNA does not usually include the teaching of sterile technique. Because of this lack of basic knowledge about asepsis, the CNA frequently has great difficulty in understanding how and why the sterile field was contaminated. As a result, over time the CNA may become less diligent in maintaining sterile technique because he or she does not fully understand the concept of preventing infection. The telemetry monitor technician has been taught to recognize potential cardiac arrhythmias but may not have a thorough understanding of what occurs within the heart during the arrhythmia. Instructors can facilitate learning for UAPs by defining complex terminology and simplifying anatomy. Based on the theory of adult learning, adults have a need to understand why an action occurs and the necessity of follow-up action in order to perform the skill at the highest level of competency.

16. The psychological response of licensed and unlicensed personnel to the same content seems to differ. Do the two groups have different personality traits?

At least one study demonstrated personality differences between registered nurses and UAPs. This study found that staff members of color, regardless of their position, demonstrated higher levels of thinking and behavioral styles related to approval, avoidance, and competitiveness. UAPs, regardless of race or ethnicity, demonstrated higher levels of thinking and behavioral styles related to dependence and opposition (see table).

THINKING/BEHAVIORAL STYLE	DESCRIPTION
Approval	Need to be accepted, seeks to please
Dependence	Follower, nonchallenging
Avoidance	Avoid conflict, self-blame for challenging
Opposition	Resists authority, critical of superiors
Competitiveness	Need to win

The evidence of these specific styles may indicate that UAPs feel a need to be seen by the registered nurse as followers who do not challenge authority. The evidence also indicates that, even though they do not directly challenge the registered nurse, UAPs may be more critical and resistant to authority—traits that have a negative effect on their ability to work effectively as a team.

Recognition of this trait allows the registered nurse to elicit appropriate input from UAPs in planning client care. By seeking input from UAPs, the registered nurse acknowledges the value of their role on the team and promotes positive recognition.

17. As budgetary constraints are enforced, the concept of cross-training often arises. Explain this concept.

Cross-training may be viewed on two distinct levels. The first level involves cross-training of staff to work in related patient care delivery areas, such as labor, delivery, recovery, and postpartum care. Other common areas may involve intensive care units and telemetry step-down units, specialty intensive care units, and postanesthesia and same-day surgery units. It is important to orient staff members to frequently practiced or high-risk procedures for each unit in which they may be assigned to work.

The second level of cross-training refers to the practice of teaching UAPs a variety of skills that are above the basic education of the CNA. Many institutions incorporate the following skills into the duties of the UAP in selected client care areas: routine activities of daily living, 12-lead electrocardiograms (EKG), interpretation of EKG strips, phlebotomy, urinary catheterization, preparation of tube feedings, respiratory treatments, priming intravenous therapy lines, and tracheostomy care. It is important that the care be provided to stable clients in whom a predictable outcome is anticipated. If the client becomes unstable, the UAP may not possess the knowledge and judgment to react appropriately, even if the UAP can perform the technical skill. The registered nurse remains responsible for delegation of skills to UAPs that do not require clinical judgment or assessment.

18. What steps should be taken in planning an orientation program that includes cross-training of staff members either to work in similar client care areas or to provide multiple technical skills?

The first step is to identify the specific duties of the new role. Guidelines from professional organizations (American Association of Critical Care Nurses, Association of Operating Room Nurses) can serve as references. It is important to verify with the state licensure board that the identified skills are within the scope of practice for the discipline. Approval may be required through institutional committees if new skills are added, especially for UAPs. Once the specific duties have been identified, specific competencies and performance criteria must be established. It is important to provide orientees with as many learning options as possible because usually they must acquire a new skill. The intended program outcome is successful demonstration of the required competencies.

19. Discuss the potential problems associated with preceptorship.

Lack of administrative support and lack of educational support are two of the most common problem areas within a preceptorship. For the preceptor to work effectively with an orientee, the manager must facilitate the following: scheduling of the preceptor to work the same shift as the new orientee, clarification of roles and responsibilities of both preceptor and orientee for other staff members, and release of the preceptor from patient care loads on the dates of orientation. Although complete release of the preceptor from patient care is not always feasible, it is unrealistic to expect that a preceptor can deliver direct patient care and effectively orient a new staff member who is providing direct care to a separate set of patients.

Lack of educational support for the preceptor creates many potential problems. The skills necessary for preceptorship are not part of basic undergraduate nursing education; therefore, unless the preceptor has been exposed to additional training, he or she will not have the essential knowledge to work effectively with the new orientee. Next, preceptors need to be knowledgeable about the CBO plan for the institution, methods of assessing learning needs, tools available for the assessment, and methods of evaluating the orientee's progress.

20. Define the role of the preceptor.

The preceptor is an experienced staff member who assists in the process of orienting new staff to a specific area or unit. The preceptor acts as a role model and educator and plays an active role in assisting the orientee in the process of socialization and role transition. The successful completion of these processes helps to reduce staff turnover and to increase retention.

21. What skills are essential for the preceptor?

The preceptor must have excellent communication skills to establish a one-on-one relationship with new staff members. The preceptor should have a working knowledge of adult learning theories and how to incorporate them into everyday clinical practice. A minimum of 1 year of clinical practice is usually expected, with at least 6 months within the institution. The preceptor must demonstrate competency in the areas in which new employees are to be evaluated and validated. Most institutions require attendance at a workshop or conference related to preceptorship before the person works with new orientees.

Sample Topics Covered in a Preceptor Workshop

Roles and responsibilities of the preceptor
Differences in orienting experienced and novice nurses
Principles of biculturism
Reality shock
Implications of learning and personality styles
Principles of adult learning theory
Effective communication and feedback
Conflict resolution
Identifying learning needs of the preceptee
Planning and implementing learning experiences
Explanation of competency-based orientation
Evaluating competency and learning performance

22. Because of budgetary constraints at my hospital, monetary rewards are not available to compensate preceptors. How can the preceptor be compensated for the additional work?

Unfortunately, not all institutions are able to provide additional funds to staff members who serve as preceptors. One of the basic criteria for being a preceptor is the sincere desire to serve in the role. Many people begin the role of preceptor because of the desire to be involved in the teaching process. The preceptor has the opportunity to practice and demonstrate teaching skills and may be rewarded at a later time with a full-time education position. It is crucial to recognize the value of the preceptor and his or her contribution to the institution. Demonstrated accomplishments in the preceptor role may be a criterion for advancement in institutions that use a clinical ladder. Additional rewards may include attendance at special events held specifically for preceptors, certificates of participation, recognition pins, special notation in the preceptor's human resources file, and recognition as "Preceptor of the Year" during annual celebrations.

23. What is the difference between an internship and an externship?

Internships were originally designed to orient the new graduate nurse and to assist in making the transition to the work setting. In the 1980s, internships became extended orientation programs designed to prepare the nurse for a specialty area within nursing practice. Today internships commonly involve highly specialized areas such a critical care, emergency care, obstetrics, and pediatrics. These types of internships usually consist of 3–6 months of orientation and clinical practice in the specialty area. Operating room internships may last as long as 12 months in some facilities. During the internship, the orientee receives classroom instruction, followed by closely monitored clinical practice with an assigned preceptor. Because the new staff member is paid a full salary during the internship, the program is expensive to operate. Most internships require the orientee to sign a contract stipulating that he or she will remain employed with the institution for a specified amount of time after the completion of the internship or repay a portion of the salary and/or course expenses.

An **externship** generally refers to a work-learn program for student nurses. The nurse externship usually is designed to allow senior nursing students to work for a facility during the summer months. Nursing students who have completed 1 year of clinical practice through an academic program are allowed to enter the externship. At the end of the summer, the nursing student returns to the academic setting and finishes the remaining year of nursing school. The intent is that the student will be given a chance to practice in the real world the skills that have been learned in school. The anticipated value to the institution sponsoring the externship is that the nursing student will return for employment at the completion of school and require less orientation.

24. Do the benefits of an internship outweigh the cost of implementing the program?

Specialty areas of nursing are currently experiencing the greatest staff shortages. Many facilities unable to recruit enough nurses to maintain staffing levels for specialty areas have decided to "grow their own nurses." The concept of educating their own staff or new graduates and providing the necessary skills for effective care is believed to promote retention. The costs of advertising positions, recruiting experienced nurses to fill the positions, and orienting experienced nurses to the facilities must be balanced against the cost-saving factors of reuse of resources, utilization of in-house teaching sources, and the value of having a pool of competently trained staff for the unit.

25. A major disadvantage to an externship is that the nursing student may not return to work for the institution at the end of the nursing program. What are some of the advantages of an externship?

Externships may be more valuable to rural hospitals that receive the majority of their graduate nurses from only 1 or 2 schools. In geographic areas of limited employment opportunities, graduate nurses may be more inclined to accept an offer of externship when they are reasonably sure that they will work for a specific hospital. An externship is designed to help nursing students use their skills in a hands-on environment. Several benefits are expected, including increased self-confidence in the clinical setting, a higher level of professional autonomy, increased self-esteem, improved time management skills, and improved performance in the remaining year of nursing school. The externship allows nursing students to work in the hospital environment with supervision to enhance decision-making skills and improve delivery of patient care before graduation.

26. Educational staff is limited within my institution. Can self-learning packets (SLPs) be used for orientation?

Many institutions use SLPs as an alternative to the usual classroom activities. The SLPs can be created or purchased to provide educational content that is specific to institutional policies and procedures. Employees must be given a designated time during work hours to complete the SLPs. Employees cannot be expected to complete orientation requirements during off-duty hours. The major advantage of SLPs is that employees can progress at their own speed.

27. Hospitals are required to orient agency staff. What suggestions can you give me to plan a low-cost agency orientation program?

The high cost of agency salaries motivates hospitals to seek the most streamlined orientation; however, they expect the same high quality of care from agency nurses. Clearly defining the content of agency orientation is important. It is helpful to work with the scheduling/office staff at the agency to determine what content is covered by the agency and to identify what hospital-specific content you need to cover. With a high volume of agency use, consider using a video tape that highlights key initiatives and issues, followed by a highly specific unit CBO that focuses on key competencies.

Appendix A: Example of a Competency-based Orientation to Maternity for Registered Nurses

At the end of the Maternal/Newborn Orientation, the professional nurse will be able to:

1. Provide family-centered care.
2. Provide for the prevention of infant abduction and respond per hospital protocol to an infant abduction.
3. Perform a systematic and thorough postpartum physical assessment based upon knowledge of normal postpartum physiological changes.
4. Provide appropriate care to the postpartum woman without complications.
5. Identify the postpartum women at risk for postpartum complications.
6. Provide care to nursing and non-nursing mothers.
7. Provide information pertaining to self and newborn care to the postpartum woman and her family based upon individual needs.
8. Perform a systematic and thorough full-term newborn physical assessment based upon knowledge of expected adaptation to extrauterine life.
9. Plan and provide care to normal full-term infants.
10. Identify the full-term infant at risk for complications.
11. Provide appropriate care to the full-term infant with complications.
12. Follow through with identified patient needs requiring intervention or referral.
13. Plan and provide care for the high-risk antepartum woman and her family.

Detailed evaluations of each of the these competencies is provided by forms listing specific knowledge and skills, each of which is observed and validated by a preceptor. Examples for competencies 2–5 are included on the following pages. All forms are reproduced with the permission of York Hospital in York, PA.

Competency 2: Provides for the prevention of infant abduction. Responds per hospital protocol to an infant abduction.

Orientee ____________________ Mentor ____________________

Critical Behavior	Self (*) Assessment	Learning Options	Method of Evaluation	Performs Independently Date/Initials
1. Identifies characteristics of a typical abductor.	________	Review P&P: "Infant Abduction Prevention and Response"	Passes exam from SLP "Infant Abduction Prevention and Response" with a score of 80% or higher	1. ________
2. Safeguards belongings that can be used by an abductor (uniform, badge).	________	View Video: "Safeguard Their Tomorrows: What Healthcare Professionals Need to Know"		2. ________
3. Performs/confirms completion of identification procedure for infants.	________			3. ________
4. Provides education to parents in prevention of infant abduction.	________	Participate in an Infant Abduction Drill		4. ________
5. Provides a safe environment for the prevention of infant abduction.	________			5. ________
6. Responds to an infant abduction per hospital protocol.	________			6. ________

(*) Self Assessment Key
1 - Knowledgeable - able to perform with confidence
2 - Knowledgeable but need practice
3 - New knowledge

Competency 3: Perform a systematic and thorough postpartum physical assessment based upon knowledge of normal postpartum physiological changes.

Orientee ____________________ Mentor ____________________

Critical Behavior	Self (*) Assessment	Learning Options	Method of Evaluation	Performs Independently Date/Initials
1. Understands normal postpartum physiological maternal adaptations.	______	View Video: AWHONN's Cross Training for Obstetrical Nursing Staff: Postpartum Care Study AWHONN's Postpartum Compendium Observes performing a postpartum assessment Practices performing a postpartum assessment	Mentor reviews charts for appropriate documentation Mentor observes the orientee assessing a postpartum woman	1. ______
2. Reviews medical record for information pertinent to the nursing plan of care: **Rh, rubella status, complications during delivery, and any other pertinent information.**	______			2. ______
3. Introduces self to patient and explains the purpose of the postpartum physical assessment.	______			3. ______
4. Provides for patient comfort and privacy by assessing need for pain relief and having patient empty her bladder.	______			4. ______
5. Obtains necessary vital signs per protocol.	______			5. ______
6. Inspects the breasts for consistency, tenderness, nipple shape, nipple integrity, and presence of colostrum or milk.	______			6. ______
7. Palpates uterine fundus noting location consistency and massages if necessary.	______			7. ______
8. Observes lochial flow for color, amount, consistency, and odor.				
9. Obtains information from patient regarding her ability to urinate independently. Notes presence of frequency, urgency, pain or the inability to empty bladder. Assesses the bladder status and catheterizes according to protocol if necessary.	______ ______			8. ______ 9. ______
10. Inspects perineum for presence and intactness of episiotomy and/or lacerations. Notes presence of erythema, ecchymosis, edema, hematoma, pain, and/or drainage in area.	______			10. ______
11. Inspects incision (Cesarean or tubal ligation) for intactness. Note presence or erythema, ecchymosis, edema, and/or drainage in area.	______			11. ______
12. Inspects intactness of rectal area noting present size, and number of hemorrhoids. Notes occurrence of last bowel movement and presence of constipation.	______			12. ______
13. Inspects extremities for presence and location of edema, redness, tenderness, and/or varicosities.	______			13. ______
14. Documents appropriately. a. Progress Notes b. Kardex c. Clinical Pathway d. OB Nursing Care Flow Sheets e. Medex	______			14. ______

(*) Self Assessment Key
1 - Knowledgeable - able to perform with confidence
2 - Knowledgeable but need practice
3 - New knowledge

Competency 4: Provide appropriate care to the postpartum woman with complications.

Orientee ____________________________ Mentor ____________________________

Critical Behavior	Self (*) Assessment	Learning Options	Method of Evaluation	Performs Independently Date/Initials
1. Receives patient report, reviews physicians' orders and patient chart.	________	Study AWHONN's Postpartum Compendium	Mentor reviews charts for appropriate documentation	1. ________
2. Initiates / follows through on plan that supports postpartum assessment and vital signs findings.	________	Review Policies & Procedures for postpartum care:	Mentor observes the orientee providing care to the postpartum woman	2. ________
3. Assesses patient's comfort level and provides for pain relief including administration and/or use of: a. pain medications - oral, IM, PCA b. ice packs c. sitz baths d. pericare measures	________	- Postpartum assessment - Medication administration - Rhogam - Rubella - Specimen collection		3. ________
4. Identifies and meets patient's psychosocial needs by utilizing referral resources within the Postpartum Home Visitation program and available Community agencies.	________	- Discharge of mother and newborn Review Mother/Baby Referral Resource Manual		4. ________
5. Provides for patient's immunization needs for Rhogam (IM) and Rubella (sc).	________			5. ________
6. Collects specimens per protocol as necessary.	________	Review self-learning packet - "The Management of Pain"		6. ________
7. Completes patient discharge per procedure.	________			7. ________
8. Documents appropriately. a. Clinical Pathway b. OB Nursing Care Flowsheets c. Progress Notes (DAO) d. Kardex e. Referrals	________	Observes peers providing care to a postpartum woman Practice providing care to a postpartum woman		8. ________

(*) Self Assessment Key
1 - Knowledgeable - able to perform with confidence
2 - Knowledgeable but need practice
3 - New knowledge

Competency 5: Identify the postpartum woman at risk for postpartum complications.

Orientee ______________________________ Mentor ______________________________

Critical Behavior	Self (*) Assessment	Learning Options	Method of Evaluation	Performs Independently Date/Initials
Postpartum Hemorrhage 1. Assesses for predisposing factors: a. previous postpartum hemorrhage b. rapid or prolonged labor c. uterine over distention due to macrosomia, multiple births, and/or polyhydramnios d. use of tocolytic and/or anesthetic agents during labor and/or delivery e. operative birth f. high parity g. intrauterine infections h. previous uterine surgery	__________	View Video: AWHONN's Cross-Training for Obstetrical Nursing Staff: Pregnancy Induced Hypertension Review March of Dimes Module: Maternal Assessment-BP Review March of Dimes Module: Maternal Assessment-urine Study AWHONN's Postpartum Compendium	Completes Identification of Postpartum Complication exam with score of 80% Mentor reviews charts for appropriate documentation Mentor observes the orientee manage the care of a postpartum woman at risk for a complication	1. __________
2. Assesses blood loss according to protocol. Keep pad count as necessary. a. Scant lochia - less than 1-inch stain on peripad within 1 hour of assessment b. Light lochia - less than 4-inch stain on peripad within 1 hour of assessment c. Moderate lochia - less than 6-inch stain on peripad within 1 hour of assessment d. Heavy lochia - saturated peripad within 1 hour of assessment	__________			2. __________
3. Assesses vital signs every 15 minutes when indicated.	__________			3. __________
4. Accurately records intake and output.	__________			4. __________
5. Plans and takes appropriate nursing actions: a. Ensure large-bore needle IV access. b. Obtains appropriate laboratory specimens. c. Massages uterus correctly. d. Anticipates need for uterotonic and pain relief medications. e. Administers appropriate IV fluids as necessary. f. Administers prescribed medications as g. Provide for emotional needs of woman and her family. h. Elevate legs to a 20 degree to 30 degree angle to increase venous return. Avoid Trendelenburg position unless ordered. i. Prepare for surgery when appropriate.	__________			5. __________
Urinary Tract Infections 1. Assess for predisposing risk factors. a. History of birth trauma, anesthesia, frequent vaginal exams, and/or catheterization.	__________			1. __________
2. Assess for appropriate signs and symptoms. a. Dysuria, frequency, low-grade fever, urgency, and/or lower pelvic pressure, back pain, chills, malaise, hematuria, and nausea and vomiting.	__________			2. __________
3. Obtain urine for analysis, culture and sensitivity.	__________			3. __________
4. Interprets lab results.	__________			4. __________
5. Administer antimicrobials as ordered.	__________			5. __________
6. Assess vital signs every 4 hours.	__________			6. __________
7. Encourages rest, adequate fluid intake, adequate diet, and frequent voiding.	__________			7. __________
8. Teach and/or reinforce appropriate perineal hygiene and hand washing.	__________			8. __________

Continued on following page

Competency 5: Identify the postpartum woman at risk for postpartum complications. *(Continued)*

Critical Behavior	Self (*) Assessment	Learning Options	Methods of Evaluation	Performs Independently
4. Initiates appropriate nursing actions: a. Assess vital signs, LOC, DTR's, urinary output, and lab data every 4 hours. b. Assesses for signs and symptoms of preeclampsia complications: 1. PP hemorrhage 2. DIC 3. Pulmonary edema 4. HELLP syndrome 5. Increased intracranial pressure 6. Intracranial hemorrhage c. Ambulate with assistance after bedrest. d. Encourage maternal-newborn attachment. e. Notifies physician appropriately.	________			Date/Initials 4. ________

(*) Self Assessment Key
1 - Knowledgeable - able to perform with confidence
2 - Knowledgeable but need practice
3 - New knowledge

BIBLIOGRAPHY

1. Abruzzese RS. Nursing Staff Development: Strategies for Success, 2nd ed. St. Louis, Mosby, 1996.
2. Alspach JG: Designing Competency Assessment Programs: A Handbook for Nursing and Health-related Professions. Pensacola, FL, NNSDO, 1996.
3. Alspach JG: The Educational Process in Nursing Staff Development. St. Louis, Mosby, 1995, pp 218–226.
4. Balcain A, et al: Action research applied to a preceptorship program. J Nurs Staff Devel 13:193–197, 1997.
5. Barczak N, Spunt D: Competency-based education: Maximize the performance of your unlicensed assistive personnel. J Contin Educ Nurs 30:254–259, 1999.
6. Benjamin BA: Level of literacy in the nurses aid population. J Nurs Staff Devel 13:149–154, 1997.
7. Craven HL, Broyles, JG: Professional development through preceptorship. J Nurs Staff Devel 12:294–299, 1996.
8. Fey MK, Miltner RS: A competency-based orientation program for new graduate nurses. J Nurs Admin 30:126–132, 2000.
9. Murray TA: Role orientation in novice home healthcare nurses. J Nurs Staff Devel 14:87, 292, 1998.
10. Nyberg DB, Campbell JL: An orientation program for unlicensed assistive personnel. Assoc Operating Room Nurse J 66:445–454, 1997.
11. Redus KM: A literature review of competency-based orientation for nurses. J Nurs Staff Devel 10:239–243, 199
12. Seago JA: Registered nurses, unlicensed assistive personnel, and organizational culture in hospitals. JONA 30:278–285, 2000.
13. Staab, S, et al: Examining competency-based orientation implementation. J Nurs Staff Devel 12:139–143, 1996.
14. Strauss J: An OR nurse internship program that focuses on retention. AORN J 66:455–463, 1997.
15. Tritak AB, et al: An evaluation of a nurse extern program. J Nurs Staff Devel 13:132–135, 1997

19. THE "C" WORD: COMPETENCY

Diann C. Cooper, MSN, RNC

Competencies—the very word can strike fear into the soul of even the most experienced educator. But it does *not* have to be this way. Assessing, maintaining, and improving competence of the staff is an important part of what staff development people do. The "what," "how," and other questions are answered in this chapter.

1. What is a competency?

The literature contains many definitions of competency and competence. Most sources define competence as the individual's capacity or potential to perform his or her job. Competency, on the other hand, is the individual's actual performance in a particular situation. A competency can be described as a single, observable, or definable skill.

2. Why are competencies important?

Competencies have been around for a long time, although not always in their current form. The idea that a person has the potential to perform and must perform at a certain level in a real situation has been around for generations. In the past, competencies ensured the passing of skills from one generation to the next. Today competencies not only describe the abilities of a particular group of people but also help to protect the public. Competence involves more than just a written checklist. It can involve licensure, certification in a specialty, and adherence to standards of practice for a particular profession (e.g., nursing, pharmacy) or an accrediting body (e.g., Joint Commission on the Accreditation of Healthcare Organizations [JCAHO]).

3. Why are they emphasized by JCAHO?

JCAHO looks at competencies in its human resources chapter. Competencies are just part of the process of maintaining a high-quality work force. Competency is the "foundation of excellent care."[5] It is important for the leaders of an organization to know that employees are able (competent) to do their jobs. Leaders should be informed on a regular basis about how well their employees have performed during the past year. This goal can be accomplished through the annual performance appraisal process and the competencies accompanying it. The report is the annual report to the board. If an employee does not demonstrate acceptable competencies, leaders should be informed of the plan of action to bring him or her up to speed. A high-quality product is produced by people who know what they are doing and do it well. In health care, this is even more important because of the product with which we deal—human lives. Employees who do not demonstrate competence can endanger the patients whom we serve.

4. Who should have competencies?

Everyone in the organization should have a job description and, as a result, competencies. The number of competencies depends on the job: the more skilled the job, the greater the number of competencies. Competencies should be developed for clinical and nonclinical staff, volunteers, contracted workers, and administrators. No need to panic—some of this work has already been done for you.

5. What do competencies look like?

A competency can be in the form of a checklist, or a special format may be developed. Competencies can be described as:

- Specific to a job title and a unit/department
- Practical (used in the everyday work world)
- Clearly and concisely written
- Demonstrable skills and activities

A competency contains two parts: a definition statement and a list of criteria. The **definition statement** explains what the person completing the competency will be able to do. For example:

- Care for the surgical patient pre- and postoperatively
- Perform preventative maintenance functions
- Perform receptionist duties

It does not contain conditions for performance and should not be detailed. Unacceptable definition statements include:

- Without access to a table of normal lab values (condition of performance), the RN identifies abnormal lab values.
- Without access to the manufacturer's recommendations, the engineer correctly locates and repairs the equipment.
- The receptionist corrects all grammatical errors without the use of a reference manual.

After the definition statement you will need to list the skills and activities that the employee must demonstrate to satisfy the competency (**list of criteria**). Each skill is written as a short sentence using action verbs (e.g., demonstrates, reads, reviews, lists, writes, locates). When you have finished the list, ask yourself if you can see the employee doing these skills. If you can—good. If you cannot (or if you need to ask more questions)—rewrite the list. Examples of lists of observable skills include the folllowing:

- Assembles the preoperative chart
- Instructs the patient on the procedure
- Administers preoperative medication
- Assesses patient postoperatively per protocol
- Describes potential postoperative complications
- Provides postoperative instructions for patient
- Describes preventive maintenance schedule for equipment X
- Demonstrates proper quality performance check on equipment X
- Documents completely, using appropriate form
- Greets customers according to customer service guidelines
- Responds to requests for information promptly
- Schedules meetings
- Types reports accurately

6. **Is there a process to follow in determining whether your staff are competent?**

Yes. JCAHO looks at four separate steps to determine competency:

1. Preemployment qualifications
2. Job preparation
3. Performance appraisal
4. Response to the appraisal

7. **Explain these steps.**

Preemployment qualifications refer to the job description and the prerequisites that people must have before they are hired. Examples include license, type of program attended, years of experience, and references. A license does not ensure competency; it simply means that the person passed a test verifying that they have the necessary knowledge. A licensed person is still expected to demonstrate the competencies of the job for which he or she has been hired.

Job preparation, which begins after the person is hired, includes orientation to the organization, department, and specific duties. Checklists and orientation competencies can be developed to assist with the process. As this process begins, you should ask the employee to review the checklist, noting any skills with which he or she is unfamiliar. This step helps to individualize the orientation.

The employee under goes an initial **performance appraisal** at the end of orientation. This step provides an opportunity to compare demonstrated job skills with the expected standard. The information contained in the performance appraisal should not be a surprise. It should be information, both positive and negative, that has already been discussed with the employee.

Step four is the **response to the appraisal**. If the appraisal indicates that the employee lacks certain competencies, an action plan is created, describing the steps to be taken to bring his or her performance up to the expected level.

8. What is an orientation or baseline competency?

Orientation competencies are determined by you and your staff for the newest members of the department. Ask yourself "What skills, knowledge, or attitudes do my newest staff members need to demonstrate before they complete orientation?" The items that you list become orientation competencies and establish a baseline for performance. Sometimes orientation includes materials that all staff review every year. These materials are called **annual competencies**.

9. How are orientation and competencies related?

Competencies are part of the orientation process. The information that a new employee receives in orientation prepares him or her to perform the job. The completion of competencies supports the achievement of orientation goals. Competency-based orientation (CBO) is a process that uses the completion of competencies to move employees from one phase of an orientation program to the next. It is highly individualized and allows experienced staff to demonstrate quickly the skills necessary to work in a particular department; it also allows new employees to learn about these skills, if needed, and to demonstrate them when they are ready. Few, if any, time restrictions exist. CBO is discussed in more detail in Chapter 18.

10. How do I identify competencies for my unit or department?

What is a competency for one department may not be for another. Choose competencies that are important for you and your staff. The following guidelines may help.

- Begin with a small group of people from your unit who represent the different levels of the clinical ladder or the different levels of experience within the department.
- Brainstorm to formulate an answer to the following question: "What items do you expect a new staff member to demonstrate by the end of orientation?"
- Write down the items.
- Look at the list and identify items that are high-risk, problem-prone, and/or low-volume.
- Reach consensus on the most important of these items that everyone must demonstrate. These become the competencies for orientation.
- Repeat this process for annual competencies. With a group of your staff, answer the question, "What high-risk, problem-prone, low-volume competencies does everyone need to demonstrate this year?"
- Develop consensus with the group as to which items have the highest priority. These are your annual competencies.
- Post both lists in your department so that everyone has a chance to comment on them. It is important for everyone to know about and support the process, if you want it to be a success. Staff members also may identify items that you missed.
- When you are ready, bring your group together again to determine the necessary format (e.g., checklist or standard format). Also choose the manner in which the competency will be assessed (e.g., game, puzzle, poster, packet, policy review, demonstration).

Some annual competencies represent topics that are too advanced to be covered during orientation. Some intensive care units (ICUs), for example, return newer staff to orientation activities after 6 months or so to cover topics that at first may have been too overwhelming. Skills such as intraaortic balloon counterpulsation may not be taught during the initial orientation to an ICU if the new person is not an experienced ICU nurse. Classes may be held later for new people to develop advanced skills, which may become part of the annual competency process.

11. Do competencies stay the same or change from year to year?

Some competencies stay the same; others should change from year to year. Orientation competencies may stay the same, because they establish a baseline for performance. Annual competencies frequently change. An activity that was problem-prone may have improved because of competency requirements and education. A new quality assurance problem may be identified, or a change in technology may require review. Perhaps a new piece of equipment has replaced an older model. It is important to review your competencies yearly and make the necessary changes. As you add new annual competencies, you should make sure that you assess whether they should become part of the orientation competencies, particularly if new equipment or new processes are involved.

12. Why look at items that are high-risk, low-volume, or problem-prone?

High-risk items can cause serious (or deadly) damage to a patient or staff member if performed incorrectly. Look at high-risk activities closely. If they are performed every day, they are considered high-volume. High-volume activities do not necessarily need to be reviewed every year, although they should be a part of your orientation program. The assumption is that you perform the activity so often that you know it well (like brushing your teeth).

Low-volume skills are not performed very often within your department, but employees still need to know how to perform them well. These skills should be reviewed at least annually. If an activity is both high-risk and low-volume, you definitely should include it in your annual review.

Problem-prone skills are the subject of incident reports or other error reporting forms or quality assurance data. These data should be reviewed regularly, because they are an excellent source of skill or knowledge deficits that become annual competencies. Near misses are also serious enough for a review.

13. What about items that are high-risk, low-volume, *and* problem-prone?

Any issue that combines all three of these criteria probably warrants an in-depth review to determine the cause of the problem as well as an educational inservice to prevent further problems. Examples may include the following:

- Cardiopulmonary resuscitation (CPR; especially high-risk on a unit where codes rarely occur)
- Administration of a particular medication (e.g., patient-controlled analgesia)
- Care of a particular age group or patient population
- Correct calculation of a drug dosage
- Checking the crash cart after a code
- Proper use of equipment (are the patients coaching your staff on its use?)

14. Discuss other sources of possible competencies.

Consider items that regulatory agencies require staff to review. JCAHO looks closely at staff education about forensic patients (prisoners), restraints, pain management, and waived testing. Lab-certifying bodies look at blood transfusion education for nursing staff. Licensing groups may require a particular number of hours reviewing information about child abuse, violence in the workplace, infection control, or Occupational Safety and Health Administration (OSHA) requirements. These items should be included on your list of competencies.

15. How do I write a competency? Should I use a particular format?

Yes and no. All competencies contain some of the same elements. However, the formats are varied. Look in the literature, and talk with other hospital educators. See what format they use, then chose one that works for you. Discuss the choice with the human resources department, which may want to standardize the form (JCAHO's "same level of care"). The completed competencies should be kept on the unit where they are accessible to the manager. The following points should be kept in mind when you write the competencies for your staff:

- Remember the KISS rule: Keep It Short and Simple. Do not make your competencies so long that they are not user-friendly. Do not repeat the entire policy in your competency. Instead, include "review of policy" as one of your criteria.
- Do not reinvent the wheel. If a checklist exists, use it.
- Use action verbs when writing statements and criteria. List observable items or changes in behaviors that are considered necessary for competency.

- Include the name of the person completing the competency, unit, and date.
- Include a spot for the criteria to be checked off by an observer.
- Include the method used to determine competence.
- At the bottom of the page, include the signature of the observer and the person observed and the date. A section for comments should be a part of the format so that the observer can make note of items that the person performs well or that need further practice. Some formats include this section at the end of the page near the signature line. Others include it as part of the body of the form, usually along the right side of the paper.

An example of a competency validation form can be found in Appendix A. Other forms can be found in the literature or obtained from regulatory bodies (e.g., JCAHO).

16. What are some of the common action verbs that I can use to write a competency?

Demonstrate	Calibrate	Check	Describe
Identify	List	Discuss	Manipulate
Modify	Examine	Explain	Summarize
Compare/contrast	Arrange	Assemble	Instruct
Perform	Coordinate	Develop	Review

17. What are the three types of competencies?

1. Skills (psychomotor)
2. Knowledge (cognitive)
3. Feelings (affective)

18. What are skills competencies? Are they difficult to write?

Skills competencies are the easiest to write; you may want to start with this type. Often skills competencies are associated with equipment. Some companies provide a competency checklist at the time of purchase or during training with a new piece of equipment. This is helpful and saves you time. Examples of skills-related competencies include:

- Use of the lift device
- Use of the defibrillator
- Programming and set-up of the cycler
- Use and programming of the IV pump
- Use of the edger/trimmer
- Use of multimedia projection system

19. How about knowledge competencies?

Knowledge-related competencies are the second easiest to write. It is usually not difficult to write down how to care for a particular patient population. Standards of care may already be written in a format that you can use. Examples of knowledge related competencies include:

- Care of the patient with myocardial infarction
- Calling a code blue team and other emergencies
- Employee's role in a fire or other disaster
- Steam sterilization process

20. What is involved in writing a competency about feelings?

The most difficult competency to write is the competency related to feelings. If this type of competency is necessary, you may want to incorporate it into a different format from the others. Often reviewing a packet with a passing score on a posttest can work. Sometimes using a video-recorded case study with a posttest can work. You can be creative with this one! Examples include:

- Care of a patient in seclusion (knowledge and feelings)
- Communication with persons of other cultures (knowledge and feelings)
- Sensitive care of a patient with a disability
- Customer service
- Teamwork

21. What are age-specific competencies?

Age-specific competencies are no different from any other competency. They simply focus on a particular age group. The purpose of an age-specific competency is to determine that direct care providers can adapt their care to the age of the patient. For example, the way you speak to a child about an IV infusion is different from how you address an adult.

22. What age groups are used for age-specific competencies?

The age groups can vary, depending on the organization and which reference you choose to use. Some hospitals use infant, child, adolescent, adult, and geriatric age groups. When you determine your age groups, make certain that you define the ages they represent. For example, some organizations may define adult as 20–49, middle adult as 50–65, older adult as 65 and above. Some may define geriatric as young old, middle old, and old old. You need to ask the direct care providers what works best for them.

23. How do you measure age-specific competency?

You may choose to define the age groups in a guideline to which staff and managers refer. This guideline is used during the performance evaluation process. It asks for specific examples of occasions when care was adapted to meet the needs of specific age groups. Written competency forms for procedures or skills also include age categories. Often specific examples of how care is to be adapted to meet the needs of various age groups can be written into the competency itself. For example, a skills competency may require evidence that a nurse can demonstrate use of a piece of equipment for different age groups. Staff are also encouraged to attend educational programs that address the needs of the different age groups that they serve. Any testing associated with these programs is evidence of age-specific knowledge (e.g., written examinations for neonatal resuscitation and pediatric advanced life support).

24. Do age-specific competencies work for staff who are not direct care providers?

Not all health care team members need to demonstrate age-specific competencies as such. Many of the items that may be considered age-specific competencies can be placed in another category, such as safety. For example, housekeepers can be asked to demonstrate age-specific care by some organizations. They can respond that they keep their cart locked and chemicals out of reach when they clean rooms on pediatric wards. This practice also can be considered a safety expectation—keep the cart locked and chemicals out of reach of any patient. The same is true of other departments. For example, making certain that teenaged patients are included in conversations about their treatment can be an age-specific expectation or a customer service expectation. The choice ultimately is made by you and your organization. Bring a group together to discuss what will work for you. Examples in the literature also may be helpful.

25. When do we refer to competencies?

Competencies are most commonly referenced during three different periods of employment: orientation, annual performance appraisal, and changes in practice, standards, or equipment. As mentioned earlier, you want to ensure that new members of your department can do certain activities (baseline or orientation competencies) before they function on their own. Annual competencies must be reviewed every year. The third occasion is whenever a change takes place. This occasion may be the easiest for some people to understand. For example, before a new piece of equipment is put to use, you make certain that staff members are trained to use it. Or perhaps you have conducted a needs assessment and plan an inservice about new pain management standards. The staff sign in and complete a posttest as a review of the material covered at the inservice. You keep the sign in and posttest on file as a competency record.

26. Where else can I find competencies?

Competencies can be found just about anywhere. When you learn how to drive a car, you take a written test and a driver's test (demonstration of skills). Both are competency tests. The next time you take a CPR class, notice how you are tested. One of the best established examples of competency testing is CPR. You receive information; you demonstrate that you can perform the skill; and you take a written test. The skills demonstration is the psychomotor competency test. The written test is the cognitive competency test. The affective aspect (feelings) is the hardest to test and is covered during the class by the instructor (as well as in the book).

27. How do I assess competence?

Competence assessment is a process that involves several people. The unit or department manager is responsible for the employees and for making certain that they are competent to perform their job. However, it is not always possible for the manager to observe personally that all staff members are doing their job. Some assistance is required. The managers need to chose the person (or people) who will verify that another person's skills are up to standard. I refer to these people as "validators."

Orientation competencies can be validated by the preceptor of the new staff member. This arrangement is ideal, because the preceptor is often close to the new employee and has the opportunity to observe his or her skills.

Annual competencies are best validated through observing direct patient care. Because this approach is not always possible, other methods can be used. Written tests can verify knowledge, demonstrations at skills stations or fairs and operating controls on equipment can validate skills, and case studies can serve as a substitute for direct patient care.

28. What is a skills fair?

A skills day or fair can be used effectively to validate the skills of the staff. A packet of information is created and distributed for review before the fair. On the day of the fair, stations are set up, and staff go from station to station to review and validate skills. A checklist is used to document the activity and stays in the mangers' personnel files. Comments about the person's abilities and the completion of the station are documented, along with any test scores.

29. What are the qualifications of a competency validator?

Validators should be experienced, senior staff members whom the managers believe to be competent, often because direct observation and prior performance appraisals consistently demonstrate that they meet or exceed the established standards. Caution the managers, however, to use objective data when choosing a validator. You never know when the manager may be asked why the person was chosen to be a validator. Be prepared.

30. How should I reassess competence? How often?

The competence of the staff should be reassessed "on a regular basis," according to the JCAHO. "Regular basis" should be determined by the hospital, often after 6 months for new employees and then annually (i.e., at the anniversary date) for everyone. Competencies can be reassessed whenever an error occurs. This decision depends on the error and may involve inservices, which all staff attend, or demonstration of a particular skill by all staff who use that skill. This process is tied to the quality assessment process. Skills stations, demonstrations, quality controls, direct observation, review of policy/procedure, posttests, inservices, case studies, videotapes, and games are among the many ways in which competencies can be reassessed. Keep in mind that you need not go looking for competencies; if there are no errors or problems, competence is assumed.

31. What methods can be used to assess competence?

Use your imagination. Be creative. Think of ways that are interesting and simple and test the information that needs to be covered. The ideas are limitless. Below are some examples:

- Use posters to review information; then test staff on the material.
- Consider using a "bulletin"; then test staff on the content (this method works well for fire safety, infection control, and other mandatories).
- Videotape assessment interviews (with the patient's permission) for annual review by the staff, with the goal of correctly identifying which diagnosis from the *Diagnostic and Statistical Manual of Mental Disorders*, 4th ed., applies to the client.

- Have your staff use the dependent lift devices to lift each other.
- Use case studies with a posttest to review lab results.
- Use a simulator to review arrhythmias.
- Consider purchasing videotapes or computer programs that can be used by many staff members. Use a test or discussion group to assess knowledge.
- Crossword puzzles and games help to vary the process.
- Treasure hunts can be used in combination with questions (i.e., answer a question, dig for a treasure).
- Exemplars can be written by staff members, describing how they handled a certain patient problem.

32. What should I do if a staff member is not competent?

Remember the difference between competence and competency. A staff member's failure to complete a competency successfully does not mean that he or she is incompetent. According to the definitions, all employees have the capacity to perform their job (competence). They may not be able to demonstrate a specific ability at this time (competency). In this case, the staff member may need additional coaching. You may need to develop a plan that outlines steps that the staff member can take to improve. The plan also may list places where staff members can go to get needed information or perhaps additional training. Often a senior staff member (validator) can provide the person with additional information so that he or she can demonstrate the competency, such as recommending a class, providing the manufacturer's instructions, or reviewing the policy. Perhaps additional experience is necessary. This strategy can be called "coaching for competence." You may need to be creative. Consider why the person is unable to complete the competency. Does the person "freeze" when asked to take a written test? Written tests are not always the best way to assess knowledge, especially in adults. Perhaps the person can demonstrate competency in another manner.

33. What about confidentiality?

It is important that you keep information about performance of competencies confidential. The only people who need to know are you, the staff person who needs to improve, the person's manager, and perhaps the human resources department.

34. How about accountability?

Staff members are accountable for their performance, and their performance is expected to be up to the standards. If their performance does not meet the standard, you must determine what the problem is. Is it a fear of testing issue? A compliance/accountability issue? Or simply a knowledge or educational issue?

35. What are the legal repercussions of being a validator?

When the validator signs a competency form, he or she is simply indicating that on a particular date specific information was reviewed or a particular skill was performed by the staff member at an expected level. It is not a guarantee of continual competence or continued acceptable performance. If, in the future, the staff person's ability to perform the skill is questioned, the signed form demonstrates that the information was reviewed and that the staff member was competent at the time of the review.

36. Who should be involved in the competency development process?

Certain key people should be involved in the development of competencies. The unit or department managers are responsible for their staff. Experienced staff members can provide valuable insight. The human resource (HR) department is responsible for the HR standards (if your organization is accredited by JCAHO). Administration is responsible for the quality of patient care, which can be affected by the competency of the staff. When you are establishing a competency program for the first time, use what you already have developed and include these people to assist you.

37. What is the relationship between competency and quality assessment?

My mother would have said, "They're kissing cousins." Competency and quality assessment are closely related. If competency is the foundation of excellent care, quality assessment is the process used to ensure that excellent care is provided. If the care is not excellent, competencies and education may be needed to improve the care provided. If the care is excellent, quality assessment continues to monitor the process.

Competencies are an important part of the work world. They are part of a continual process to help ensure that the organization provides high-quality care to its customers and patients. By taking time to reflect on the unit or department, you can identify what skills, knowledge and attitudes you expect your staff to demonstrate. High-risk, problem-prone, and/or low-volume items help you to keep a finger on the abilities of your staff and to identify when additional support is needed. Competencies do not have to cause fear. They can be a vital part of a well-planned staff development and quality assurance program.

Appendix A: Hamot Medical Center Competency Validation Form

Name ______________________________ Title ______________________________

Baseline: __________ Annual: __________

Age groups served (check all that apply):

☐ infant ☐ pediatric ☐ adolescent ☐ adult ☐ geriatric

TITLE OF COMPETENCY

Skill	Verbalize	Demonstrate	Met	Comments
Upon completion, the nurse will demonstrate competence in:				
1.				
2.				
3.				
4.				
5.				
6.				
7.				
8.				
9.				
10.				
11.				
12.				
13.				
14.				
15.				

Validator's Initials: ______ Signature/Title: ______________________________

Employee's Signature: ______________________________ Date: ______________

Used with permission of Hamot Medical Center, Erie, PA.

BIBLIOGRAPHY

1. Alspach JG: The Educational Process in Nursing Staff Development. St. Louis, Mosby, 1995.
2. American Society for Health Care Education and Training of the American Hospital Association: Competency Assessment: Challenges and Opportunities for Health Care Educators. Chicago, American Hospital Association, 1992.
3. del Bueno DJ, Altano R: Competency-based education: No magic feather. Nurs Manage 4:48–53, 1984
4. Hall JL: Developing meaningful age-appropriate competencies for clinical services. J Nurs StaffF Devel 6:241–250, 1999.
5. Joint Commission Resources: Staff competency is foundation of excellent care. J Commission Perspect 3:4, 1994
6. Kobs A: Competence: The shot heard around the nursing world. Nurs Manage 28:10–12, 1997.
7. Lawlinger SJ: Competency-based orientation program for a surgical intensive therapy unit: Parts 1–4. Crit Care Nurse 4:36–44, 52–60, 20–32, 44–55 , 1991.
8. McConnell EA: Competence and competency: Keeping your skills sharp. Nursing 9:2, 4, 1998.
9. McLagan P: Competencies. Training Dev 51:40–47, 1997.
10. Wright D: The Ultimate Guide to Competency Assessment in Healthcare. Eau Claire, WI, PESI Healthcare, LLC, 1998.

20. THE MANDATORIES

Kristen L. *O'Shea*, MS, RN, *and Linda* S. *Smith*, MS, DSN, RN

1. How does education become mandatory?

Nurses and other health care workers need continuing education to maintain a current practice. With the current explosion of new knowledge, technology, and treatment modalities, it is important that continuing education be available to staff. Because continuing education is given such a high level of importance, many different agencies and governing bodies have believed it necessary to mandate certain education for nurses and health care workers.

2. What is meant by "the mandatories"?

When staff development educators use the term *mandatories*, they generally are referring to life-safety issues that are evaluated by the Joint Commission for Accreditation for Healthcare Organizations (JCAHO) and the Occupational Safety and Health Administration (OSHA). Staff must know what to do in the case of an emergency and how to protect themselves and others from injury. In an effort to ensure that everyone knows what to do, many health care organizations group subjects such as fire safety, back safety, infection control, electrical safety, and radiation and magnet safety into an annual educational offering. These competencies are reviewed in question 6.

3. What other types of group may impose mandatories?

Many states have a continuing education requirement for licensure (see question 12 for a complete listing). In addition, most specialty certification boards require continuing education hours in lieu of an examination for renewal of certification. For example, to renew critical care certification (CCRN), the nurse must supply evidence of 100 continuing education recognition points over a 3-year period. Finally, hospitals and health care organizations often have policies requiring continuing education as a job expectation (see Appendix A for an example).

4. How can I identify what is required?

This determination can be quite tricky. You want to see what is required by JCAHO, OSHA, the Health Care Financing Administration (HCFA), and your state department of health. Other requirements may be based on specialty. In Pennsylvania, for example, a hospital must submit evidence of continuing education to the Pennsylvania Trauma Systems Foundation to maintain credentials as a level 1 trauma center. The foundation mandates that each registered nurse within a unit that provides care to trauma patients must have an accredited trauma nursing course, advanced cardiac life support (ACLS), and eight trauma-related contact hours. In addition, specialty certifications are mandated for at least half of the registered nurses in the emergency department and intensive care unit.

One word of advice: go to the manuals for each of the accrediting bodies that evaluates your institution. Read for yourself to find out what is required. People tend to create more work than is needed by reacting to other people in their institutions who say, "JCAHO requires this," when a little research reveals that JCAHO has no such requirement.

Another interesting twist is that the accrediting bodies evaluate you against what you say is your policy. If the institution has a policy that all staff should receive information about a certain topic on an annual basis, you will be evaluated to see whether you followed through.

5. What agencies affect mandatory staff education?

The mission of **JCAHO** is "to continuously improve the safety and quality of care provided to the public through the provision of health care accreditation and related services that support performance improvement in health care organizations." You can find JCAHO standards on its website: www.jcaho.org.

The **Healthcare Facilities Accreditation Program (HFAP)** accredits osteopathic organizations.

The mission of **OSHA** is to ensure safe and healthful workplaces in America. OSHA mandates training that reinforces how employees can protect themselves from bloodborne pathogens, back injury, and other occupational hazards. OSHA maintains a large website at www.osha.gov.

HCFA recently was renamed the Center for Medicare and Medicaid Services (CMS). It regulates Medicare and Medicaid spending and ensures that hospitals follow standards related to confidentiality and restraint use. The website can be found at www.cms.hhs.gov or at www.hcfa.gov.

Another important player is your **state department of health**, which maintains regulatory oversight of health care organizations. You need to request these regulations, which vary from state to state.

6. Give examples of life/safety issues that need to be addressed.

Hospital Accreditation Standards: Life/Safety Issues

1. Staff can describe or demonstrate:
   - Safety risks in the hospital environment
   - Reporting procedures for incidents involving property damage and occupational illness or injury to patients, staff, or visitors
   - Actions to eliminate, minimize, or report safety risks
   - Hospital-specific fire evacuation routes
   - Their specific roles and responsibilities at a fire's point of origin
   - Their specific roles and responsibilities away from a fire's point of origin
   - Use and functioning of fire alarm systems, when required
   - Their specific role and responsibilities in preparing for building evacuation
2. Personnel can describe or demonstrate:
   - Location and proper use of equipment for evacuating or transporting patients to refuse areas during a fire
   - Building compartmentalization procedure for containing smoke and fire
3. Personnel in security-sensitive areas of the environment of care can describe or demonstrate:
   - Processes for minimizing security risks
   - Reporting procedures for security incidents involving patients, visitors, personnel, and property
   - Emergency procedures for security incidents involving patients, visitors, staff, and property
4. Personnel who manage or have contact with hazardous materials and waste can describe or demonstrate:
   - Procedures and precautions for selecting, handling, storing, using, and disposing of hazardous material and waste spills or exposures
   - Health hazards of mishandling hazardous materials and waste
   - Reporting procedures for hazardous materials and waste spills or exposures
5. Personnel who participate in the emergency management plan can describe and demonstrate:
   - Their roles and responsibilities for emergency preparedness, as applicable
   - Their roles and past participation in organization-wide drills
   - Back-up communication system during disasters and emergencies
   - How to obtain supplies and equipment during disasters or emergencies
6. Medical equipment users can describe or demonstrate:
   - Capabilities, limitations, and special applications of equipment
   - Operating and safety procedures for equipment use
   - Equipment procedures in the event of an equipment failure
   - Reporting procedures for equipment problems and failures or user errors
7. Medical equipment maintainers can demonstrate or describe:
   - Knowledge and skills necessary to perform maintenance responsibilities
   - Processes for reporting equipment management problems or failures and user errors
8. Utility system users can describe or demonstrate:
   - Processes for reporting utility system management problems or failures and user errors
   - Utility system capabilities, limitations, and special applications

Continued on following page

Hospital Accreditation Standards: Life/Safety Issues (Continued)

- Emergency procedures in the event of a system failure
- Location and use of emergency shut-off controls
- Whom to contact in emergencies

9. Personnel can describe or demonstrate:
   - Safe clean-up of blood/body fluid spills
   - Appropriate use of personal protective equipment
   - How to protect themselves and others from bloodborne, airborne, and contact transmissions
   - Proper body mechanics

Used with permission of Wellspan Health, York, PA.

7. This information seems quite important. Why does everyone groan when I mention mandatories?

Mandatories are required by a variety of state and national agencies. Staff rebel against the idea of imposed requirements. Much of the information is dry and a bit boring. In addition, staff may feel that this education is not necessary. For these reasons, staff and educators groan. Nowhere, however, does the list of requirements in question 6 say, "This information must be provided yearly in a boring educational session." The agencies focus on outcomes, which means that your staff knows what to do in an emergency and how to keep themselves safe. Many organizations have massive required education days that teach the same information year after year. You need to evaluate this approach in your organization.

8. What can I do to revive mandatory life/safety education at my hospital?

First of all, adults need to know that the information is important to them. In some ways, the terrorists' activities of September 11, 2001, have created a new interest in the life/safety topics. Build on that interest. Our hospital offered its annual "Fire School" the week after September 11. We had over 1200 participants. People suddenly saw a reason for knowing what to do.

Too often mandatory education is on auto-pilot. You should keep the information fresh and timely. Brain storm the numerous possibilities for mandatory education. Try to offer many different options for people who have a variety of different learning styles and preferences. Find fun, fast ways to get the information to people. Suggestions include the following:

- Safety fair
- Chamber of horrors (many different hazards are displayed; people who identify the most hazards win a prize)
- Computer-based training
- Unit-based safety days with scenarios
- Bathroom learning (information posted on door)
- Mock drills
- Table top drills
- Self-learning packets
- Safety bulletin boards
- Unit-based education that focuses on use of concepts in specific clinical areas

9. Our hospital requires several different mandatory education modules for all employees (e.g., fire safety, infection control, electrical safety). We offer many different options for education, some of which are even fun and easy. Still our compliance is less than 80%. What else can I do to encourage participation?

1. Work with your managers to ensure that they are setting the expectation that all staff will complete the mandatory education. Management support is critical. When managers set the expectation, compliance is higher.

2. Provide monthly compliance monitors to the managers with plenty of positive reinforcement for the areas with the highest compliance. Adults are competitive. In addition, with accurate data, managers are better able to do their jobs.

3. If your hospital has a weekly or monthly newsletter, write regular updates monitoring completion of the annual education requirements.

10. What is my role in relation to JCAHO?

To some extent, your role obviously depends on your health care institution and its structure. Whether you have a formal or informal role in the JCAHO visit, you should up to date with JCAHO standards and hot issues. Staff education will be necessary for many of these hot issues.

You can help prepare staff for a JCAHO visit in many creative ways. You can play games to assess knowledge ("Who Wants To Be A Millionaire" works well. Give $100,000 candy bars as prizes). You can prepare posters to increase awareness and knowledge. You can become a "mock surveyor" and visit the units to ask questions and look for problems. As an objective third party, you may be able to see problems that others who are on the unit daily may not see.

During the JCAHO visit, you may be asked to sit in on one or more of the interviews. It is helpful to have an educator present during the human resources interview as well as the nursing leadership interview.

11. What is HIPPA?

HIPPA is the Health Insurance Portability and Accountability Act of 1996. It is in the process of being implemented by the year 2004. Title II of the act deals with fraud and abuse and specifically the confidentiality of health care information. Staff need to be educated about the importance of HIPPA and confidentiality as well as about new types of electronic measures that will be implemented as a result of HIPPA.

12. Summarize some states' continuing education requirements for licensure of nurses.

STATE	NUMBER OF CONTACT HOURS	PERIOD OF TIME (YR)
Alabama	24	2
Alaska	30	
California	30	2
Delaware	30	2
Florida (must include 1 hr in domestic violence, 1 hr in HIV/AIDS)	25	2
Iowa	45	3
Kansas	30	2
Kentucky (2 hr in AIDS, 3 hr in domestic violence; medication safety within 3 years of graduation)	30	2
Louisiana	15	1
Massachusetts	15	1
Michigan	25	2
Minnesota	24	2
Nebraska	20	2
Nevada	30	2
New Hampshire	30	2
New Mexico	30 (or certification)	2
Ohio	24	2
Texas	20	2
Utah	30	2
West Virginia	30	2
Wyoming	20	2

13. What are the hot clinical issues? Why may they become subjects in mandatory education within a health care organization?

A number of clinical issues are important for accreditation by JCAHO, HCFA/CMS, and others. All clinical staff should be aware of these issues and attempt to provide the best possible care. In some cases, hospitals make education mandatory to achieve compliance and ensure that the staff is well versed in certain topics. In addition, some states require specific topics. For example, as noted in question 12, some states require annual education in domestic violence and AIDS/HIV. Other hot topics include:

- Cultural competence
- Pain management (new JCAHO standards in 2001)
- Age-specific care
- Use of restraints (continually revised standards from JCAHO and HCFA/CMS)
- Fall prevention
- Medical and medication error reduction

You should ensure that these topics are thoroughly discussed and create a plan for their incorporation into clinical education. It is helpful to work with a hospital or system-wide task force or committee to:

- Identify the importance of the topic
- Plan and implement programming, including educational offerings
- Identify possible quality assurance indicators/data for study
- Evaluate effectiveness

"HOT TOPIC" INITIATIVES: CULTURAL COMPETENCE AND PAIN MANAGEMENT

14. Why is culturally competent health care such an important staff development priority?

In addition to JCAHO and government mandates, culturally competent health care is important because of the growing diversity of staff, communities, and clients. All persons, regardless of race, religion, or ethnic background, have a cultural heritage that should be understood and respected. Culture is learned and greatly affects how we perceive and maintain health, how we interact with societies and environments, and how we perceive and interact with the health care industry. Culturally incompetent care has negative effects on morbidity and mortality rates. Culturally competent care moves clients forward toward improved quality of life and health status. To be effective, efficient providers, health care staff must be able to bridge the cultural gaps among fellow staff members and clients.

15. Why is diversity such a big issue?

The United States and the health care profession are increasingly more diverse. By the year 2050 it is expected that the minority population will grow from 28% (1998) to 47%. This growth rate includes an estimated 820,000 immigrants per year. The dramatic increase is due to immigration and a higher birth rate, on average, among minority groups, even though they have higher morbidity and mortality rates. According to 2001 data from the Health Resources Services Administration (HRSA), the registered nurse (RN) population is also becoming more diverse. Of the 2,696,540 currently licensed RNs, 4.4% are older than 64, 5.9% are male, and 12.3% report a nonwhite ethnic background. With an aging, increasingly varied workforce (the average age of RNs is 45.2 years), staff development professionals need to discover new and creative ways of teaching, learning, and implementing culturally competent care.

16. How do I measure and document cultural competence among health care staff?

The measurement and documentation of cultural competence are critically important. Precious little empirical research has been done on the identification of cultural competence. Three valid and reliable tools for measurement of cultural competence have been developed and are available from their authors: The Cultural Self-Efficacy Scale (CSES),[2] Cultural Knowledge-Based Questions,[9] and the Cultural Attitude Scale–Modified.[3,9]

With the consultation of one or more cultural competence experts, you also may be able to formulate your own set of questions and answers. To do so, you need to separate questions (one stem, four distracters, multiple choice) into four categories: general cultural competence information and specific information regarding the three most common cultural groups that your staff encounter. Develop reliability and validity data by asking for feedback from cultural competence experts (do these questions assess cultural competence?), educators (are these questions worded appropriately?), and staff (what is confusing or difficult about this tool?). You also may test and retest the questions on a representative sample of staff members. You are looking for a representative number of questions that will take no longer than about 20 minutes to complete. You also may choose to run statistical analyses. The aim, of course, is to ensure that questions discriminate between cultural competence and incompetence. Be sure to record all of your tool-development steps.

17. How should I plan a cultural competence program?

Once you have created or obtained a valid and reliable cultural competence tool, the first step in developing a cultural competence program is to administer the tool to your staff. If you promise complete anonymity and ask only for job titles but no names, you will have better compliance. Before the multiple choice questions, create a section on the examination that asks staff to:

- Describe cultural competence and its importance to their work
- Explain their short- and long-term needs for development of cultural competence
- Identify desired program format

The results of these multiple choice and fill-in answers are important to program content and design and serve to answer several questions:

- Which job titles have the lowest/highest scores?
- Which content areas seemed difficult/easy?
- What are staff perceptions and needs?
- What are staff expectations for cultural competence teaching/learning?

18. What needs to be included in a facility-wide cultural competence workshop?

One well-researched cultural competence program consisted of an 8½-hour workshop that began and ended with the administration of a reliability/validity measure. This method is used to validate an improved level of cultural competence among staff. Smith[11] used an intensive educational program that included 8.5 hours of teaching/learning with PowerPoint, formal content, simulations, role modeling, demonstrations, and return demonstrations. It was based on the pragmatic Giger-Davidhizar Transcultural Assessment Model and Theory,[4] which is easy to describe and implement clinically.

19. Whom should I invite as guest speakers for cultural competence issues?

It is never appropriate to ask any individual to speak on behalf of his or her culture. However, you may wish to conduct focus groups composed of ethnically similar members to ask their opinion about possible guest speakers and expert health care culture brokers. You also want to seek cultural competence experts within your community.

One important source is the local university or community college. Because nursing school curricula must include cultural competence, faculty working for your nearest nursing school are excellent resources. Even if they do not perceive themselves as culturally competent, they almost always have a person or persons to recommend. Faculty also can recommend print and media resources. They may even make these resources available to you for zero cost and effort.

Do not restrict yourself to nursing resources. Cultural competence is an international initiative in industry and business.

20. As a staff development professional, what can I do to improve cultural competence among all health care staff?

For practicing health care staff, an important source of cultural competence information is staff development. Thus, your role in improving cultural competence facility-wide is an important one. One class or program, however, cannot create an environment for ongoing improvement of culturally competent care. Below are a few suggestions for a continued effort and emphasis on cultural competence among your staff.

- Journal clubs that meet monthly to discuss culturally related media items and events.
- Monthly organized potluck dinners with a cultural dish and theme. Members of the target culture are given the opportunity to cook and share.
- A session during each staff meeting to focus on culture-related problems among staff and clients. Ideally, these sessions will evolve into formally presented case studies.
- Quarterly inservice related to cultural competence and based on needs assessments.
- An anonymous suggestion box to discuss cultural incongruence between staff and clients.
- Facility-wide policies and procedures that demonstrate mission, importance, and commitment to culturally competent environments and care.
- Staff development professionals who sit on all or most facility-wide committees dealing with care processes. Examples include policy and procedures, ethics, risk management, and marketing.
- A cultural competence corner in each newsletter. Items for this dedicated space could be solicited from all staff.
- Include cultural competence as a job requirement for all levels of care; include cultural competence as a required parameter within all performance evaluation tools and discussions.

21. Why is pain management such an important priority for staff development?

Recent attention to pain management is as a result of new JCAHO standards published in 2000 and 2001. JCAHO identified pain management as an important aspect of care. In addition, the commission found that undertreatment of pain is a major problem in health care. JCAHO developed standards that were consistent with pain management guidelines developed by the Agency for Healthcare Research and Quality and the American Pain Society. These new standards affect not only hospitals but also ambulatory care, behavioral health, home care, long-term care, long-term care planning, and health care network organizations. Pain management has been added to six of the standards chapters:

1. Patient Rights and Ethics: recognizes the right of patients to appropriate assessment and management of pain.
2. Assessment of Patients: requires assessment of the presence, nature, and intensity of pain in all patients.
3. Care of Patients: requires establishment of policies and procedures that support appropriate pain management (e.g., appropriate prescribing, use of patient-controlled analgesia).
4. Education: requires education of patients and families about effective pain management.
5. Continuum of Care: identifies the need for symptom management to be addressed as part of the discharge planning process.
6. Improving Organization Performance: requires that pain management be incorporated into your organization's performance measurement and improvement program.

22. How do I measure pain management competence among health care workers?

Pain management competence can be measured in many different ways. Staff attitudes and knowledge regarding pain can be measured via a question and answer test. Chart audit and clinical outcomes can also provide valuable information. For example, using a chart audit, you could determine whether staff are using pain scales for assessment of pain.

A national study of acute pain management, Total Quality Pain Management, TQPM, is accepted as one of the performance measurement systems in the ORYX initiative for JCAHO. This national database provides hospitals with the ability to compare their own data against national pain management data. This national initiative is based on patient satisfaction. Patient satisfaction surveys can provide you with great information about how nurses and other staff respond to complaints of pain and treat pain.

23. What can a pain management task force do?

A pain management task force helps to champion the importance of the topic. A multidisciplinary group is essential. The membership should include nurses, pharmacists, physicians, and clinical support departments. The group must become knowledgeable about pain management issues and the JCAHO pain management standards and should be responsible for an action plan that includes staff education, assessment of staff competency, collection and interpretation of data, development of ongoing programming, and identification of ongoing needs and issues.

24. As a staff development educator, what can I do to improve pain management competence among all health care staff?

You should work in conjunction with the pain management task force or group within your organization. Below is a list of ideas:

- Develop computer-based awareness training for all staff. The associated competency test should be mandatory for all clinical staff.
- Implement a Pain Day Fair.
- Include speakers, raffles, quizzes (baseline information), and puzzles.
- Initiate a series of inservices that discuss important pain management issues, including update on complementary therapies, barriers to pain management, treatment principles, and new technologies.
- Consider implementation of a pain resource nurse program, which should be designed to educate a small number of nurses to act as resource persons on their clinical units. You can become involved in the planning of the educational offerings that support this program.
- Provide signs in the clinical areas making patients and staff aware that pain management is important.
- Provide medication resources for clinical use (paper form or via computer) with new medications and equivalencies.
- Publicize pain management initiatives and best practices in your hospital.
- Use quality improvement data to pinpoint areas of improvement.
- In association with clinical experts, develop a pain management algorithm as a resource for staff.

Appendix A: Sample Nursing Education Requirements Policy

YORK HOSPITAL — NURSING POLICY AND PROCEDURE

DATES: Effective September 1995
Reviewed June 2001
Revised June 2001

TITLE: NURSING EDUCATION REQUIREMENTS

I. **PURPOSE:**
To outline staff education requirements which support and maintain staff competency.

II. **POLICY STATEMENT:**
The Nursing Education requirements outlined in this policy support the competency assessment process. Education requirements are established to maintain and improve competency on an ongoing basis.

III. **EQUIPMENT:**
Database
Registrar Training Administration System
HRIS Employee Education Record

IV. **PROCEDURE:**

A. Required Education Program for Staff

1. The accumulation of contact hours is the responsibility of the nurse as outlined in the clinical ladder.
   a. Within the course of one year RNs and LPNs are required to have the following CEUs.

	Full Time	*Part Time*
LPN	20	10
CN I	20	10
CN II	30	15
CN III	40	20

   b. See unit-specific Policy and Procedures for additional contact hour requirements.
2. Programs attended may be sponsored by the hospital or other health agencies/organizations. The hospital offers a variety of educational opportunities from inservices to self learning modules and computer based training.
3. Documented evidence of attendance or participation for programs not presented or coordinated by Education Services must be presented to the appropriate manager for approval for inclusion in the employee's educational file.
   a. A copy of the certificate of attendance should be sent to Education Services in a timely fashion following the program.
4. A printout is available in the Registrar Database of an individual's ongoing education activity by calling Education Services
5. Contact hours may be accumulated according to the following criteria: See attached.

B. Required Education Programs for ALL CLINICAL Staff

1. Continuing Education Programs have been mandated for attendance by nursing personnel. Nursing personnel are required to attend the following programs.

Program	*Frequency*	*Target Audience*
Personal Safety Training • Electrical Safety • Fire Safety • Radiation Safety • Standard Precautions: Blood and Body Fluids • Transmission Precautions Airborne and Contact • Back Safety	q 1 year	all levels
BCLS	q 2 year	all levels
Fire School	q 3 year	all levels
Restraints	q 1 year	all levels

2. Other programs may be required as the need arises.

C. Required education for staff on *monitored/telemetry* areas:
   1. *Expectations:*
      a. *Professional Registered Nurses:* must successfully complete the EKG I offered through Education Services; will attend the first available course after employment on the unit. Until that time, staff will be teamed with a nurse who has successfully completed the course in order to facilitate patient care. A computer-based EKG is available as a self learning option.
      b. *Licensed Practical Nurse and Monitor Technicians:* must successfully complete the Rhythm Recognition course offered through Education Services; will attend the first available course after employment on the unit. Until that time, staff will be teamed with an individual who has successfully completed the course in order to facilitate patient care.
      c. *Conditions:*
         1) Staff who have previously taken a comparable course may challenge the EKG with Rhythm Recognition course after evaluation by the nurse manager and course instructor, and by successfully passing the final exam within three months of employment.
         2) If unable to successfully challenge, staff will enroll in the first available course.
         3) Staff members who do not successfully complete the course by achieving the required average on quizzes and passing the final exam, will be provided with an additional six weeks to prepare to retake the necessary quizzes and/or final exam.
         4) Staff who fail to pass the course with this second attempt will have 30 days to find employment in another position not requiring telemetry. If this individual is not able to find another position he/she will be terminated. The individual will be eligible to apply for other available positions in the WellSpan Health–York Hospital, for which he/she is qualified.

D. Intensive Care/Transitional Care Staff
   In addition to A to C all staff members employed in the ICU/TCU environment need to maintain the following educational requirements.
   1. RNs must obtain BCLS within their orientation period and ACLS within one year of hire date. BCLS/ACLS status must be maintained.
   2. The Critical Care Course/Transitional Care Course must be successfully completed at the next available course offered or the RN must successfully complete the challenge examine three months of hire date. A minimum of 80% must be obtained to pass course.
   3. A minimum of 25% of continuing education contact hours must be critical care related topics for ICU staff.
   4. RNs employed in Trauma Surgical ICU must take the CCRN test within two years of employment or as soon as eligible.
   5. TSICU RNs need to successfully complete PALS at the first available course.
   6. RNs employed in Open Heart ICU must complete the Open Heart ICU class at the first available class offered.
   7. Staff in CCU/MICU must attend a four hour introduction to Balloon pumping class.
   8. RNs on 3 South and STCU must attend the Open Heart Transitional Class.
   9. If education requirements are not successfully completed within established timeframe based on frequency of course offerings a employee will be requested to transfer from the ICU/TCU.
   10. *Trauma Requirement:* See Trauma Manual for educational requirements.
   11. *PRN Staff*
       a. Must complete nursing orientation by Education Services.
       b. Must complete mandatory program on page 2-B, on annual basis.
       c. RNs in the ICU/TCU area must successfully complete EKG exam and maintain current BCLS and ACLS certification.
       d. ICU RNs need to pass the Critical Care Challenge exam with an 80% or have current CCRN certification.
       e. Must meet requirements of the appropriate areas.

E. Nursing Education Programs for Students
   1. Nursing Leadership consults and cooperates with the faculty of the nursing education program affiliating with the hospital in providing clinical experience for nursing students.

2. Such experience must be in compliance with the philosophy and objectives of the hospital and the objectives of the school curriculum.
3. The nursing staff serve as a clinical resource and as role models for the students.
4. The student while in clinical practice is the responsibility of the clinical instructor and the patient remains the responsibility of the hospital

V. **DOCUMENTATION:**
Employee Education Record

VI. **APPLIES TO: PERSONS PERMITTED TO PERFORM:**

RN	✓	
LPN	✓	
Other	✓	All other health care providers as defined within their scope of practice.

VII. **AREA PERFORMED:**
All patient care areas.

VIII. **REFERENCES/RESOURCES:**
WellSpan Health–York Hospital Human Resources Department

Reprinted with permission of York Hospital, York, PA.

BIBLIOGRAPHY

1. Apgar C: Making it count: Key factors to consider when assessing continuing professional education offers. J Trauma Nurs 6:6–14, 1999.
2. Bernal H, Froman R: Influences on the cultural self-efficacy of community health nurses. J Transcult Nurs 4:24–31, 1993.
3. Bonaparte BH: Ego defensiveness, open-closed mindedness, and nurses' attitude toward culturally different patients. Nurs Res 28:166–172, 1979.
4. Giger JN, Davidhizar RE (eds): Transcultural Nursing: Assessment and Intervention, 3rd ed. St. Louis, Mosby, 1999.
5. Heye ML, Goddard LR: Teaching pain management: How to make it work. J Nurs Staff Devel 15:27–35, 1999.
6. Health Resources and Services Administration [HRSA], HHS, Bureau of Health Professions, Division of Nursing: The Registered Nurse Population: National Sample Survey of Registered Nurses 2001. Available at http://phpr.hrsa.gov.
7. Joint Commission: Pain Assessment and Management: An Organizational Approach. Oakbrook Terrace, IL, Joint Commission on Accreditation of Healthcare Organizations, 2000.
8. Population Reference Bureau: America's Racial and Ethnic Minorities. Population Bulletin, 1999. Available at http://www.prb.org/pubs/population_bulletin/bu54-3/part3.htm.
9. Rooda LA: Knowledge and Attitudes of Nurses toward Culturally Diverse Patients. Unpublished doctoral dissertation, Purdue University, West Lafayette, Indiana, 1990.
10. Sayers M, et al: No need for pain. J Healthcare Qual 22:10–15, 2000.
11. Smith LS: Evaluation of an educational intervention to increase cultural competence among registered nurses. J Cult Diversity 8:50–63, 2001.

For state continuing education requirements, contact your state board of nursing or refer to www.slackinc.com/allied/jcen/2001ce1.htm .

21. MAKING SENSE OF LIFE SUPPORT COURSES

Daryl Boucher, RN, MSN, EMT-P, *and John* L. *LaBrie,* RN, BSN

1. Summarize the history of life support courses.

In 1966, the first of six national emergency cardiovascular care conferences took place. At that time the National Research Council/National Academy of Sciences officially endorsed cardiopulmonary resuscitation (CPR) for medical professionals. Eight years later (1973) at the second national conference, CPR was approved for the lay public. In 1979, guidelines and standards for adult and pediatric basic life support (BLS) and advanced cardiac life support (ACLS) were approved. Early defibrillation was first emphasized in 1985. At the fifth national conference in 1992, past recommendations were reviewed and reaffirmed using scientific and clinical data.

At the latest conference, which took place in 2000, guidelines based on international science and produced by international resuscitation experts were adopted. Authorities in cardiology and emergency cardiac care reviewed various evidence-based research. These studies reflected the areas of technique, procedures, and pharmacology pertaining to BLS, CPR, ACLS, neonatal advanced life support (NALS), and pediatric advance life support (PALS).

2. What types of cardiovascular care courses has the American Heart Association (AHA) developed?

Seven different types of BLS courses are now available at the basic level. In addition, several more courses are available at the advanced levels.

American Heart Association Programs

COURSE	MANUAL NEEDED	TARGET AUDIENCE	SKILLS LEARNED	EDUCATIONAL APPROACH	TESTING METHOD
CPR for Family and Friends	CPR for Family and Friends	General public	Phone 911, mouth-to-mouth rescue breathing, 1 rescuer CPR, and relief of foreign body in unresponsive victim	Brief course; concise video, then practice approach	Skill demonstration and group practice; participation card is given
Heart-Saver CPR	Heart-Saver CPR	Credentialed lay responders such as police, security, firefighters, lifeguards	Phone 911, rescue breathing using barrier, 1 rescuer adult CPR, and relief of foreign body obstruction; pediatric and infant sequence modules are included but optional	Watch, then practice video instruction, scenarios, and peer practice	Annotated written exam and skills in foreign body removal, CPR, and rescue breathing
Heart-Saver AED	Heart-Saver CPR	Lay responders as above, but with capability of performing automatic external defibrillation (AED)	Phone 911, rescue breathing using barrier device, 1 rescuer CPR, safe and accurate use of AED, and relief of foreign body obstruction in responsive victim; child and infant sequences are included but optional	Watch, then practice video instruction, scenarios, and peer practice; instructor-led, hands-on scenario practice	Practical evaluation of all skills, written exam using annotated format

Continued on following page

American Heart Association Programs (Continued)

COURSE	MANUAL NEEDED	TARGET AUDIENCE	SKILLS LEARNED	EDUCATIONAL APPROACH	TESTING METHOD
Heart-Saver FACTS	FACTS	Lay responders as above, with capability of performing CPR, AED, and first aid	Phone 911, rescue breathing, including use of barrier device, 1 rescuer CPR, safe and accurate use of AED, relief of foreign body obstruction, how to assess ill or injured victim, bleeding control and bandaging, and extremity immobilization	Lecture with slides plus video (watch, then practice), instructor-led, scenario-based practice	Practical evaluation of all skills and written exam
BLS for Health-care Providers	BLS for Health-care Providers	Licensed and certified health care providers (e.g., nurses, paramedics, physicians)	Activation of 911, rescue breathing with mouth to barrier and bag-valve mask; 1 and 2 rescuer CPR for adult, infant, and child; use of AED, relief of foreign body in unresponsive and responsive victims of any age	Video (watch, then practice), scenario and peer practice	BLS skills evaluation and written exam
	Fundamentals of BLS for Health-care Providers	Nonlicensed and certified health care providers (e.g., phlebotomists, office staff, dental assistants)			
Heart-Saver CPR in Schools	Heart-Saver CPR in Schools	Middle and high school students	Phone 911, rescue breathing, 1 rescuer CPR, relief of foreign body obstruction, safe and correct use of AED	Watch, then practice video, case scenario practice	Evaluation of all skills is optional but suggested
Mass CPR	CPR for Family and Friends	Training of large number of community members who do not require an official credential	Phone 911, rescue mouth-to-mouth breathing, 1 rescuer CPR, and relief of foreign body obstruction in responsive victim	Hundreds of people are trained simultaneously using video (watch, then practice), scenario with peer practice	Scenario with peer practice; generally no cards are issued
Pediatric Advanced Life Support (PALS)	Provider Manual for Pediatric Advanced Life Support (PALS)	Health care professionals who care for infants and children	Early identification of respiratory failure and shock, advanced airway management, CPR, vascular access and medication administration, intraosseous access, and post-resuscitation management	Case scenarios, skills stations with demonstration and peer practice, small group discussion	Annotated written exam and skills station evaluation
Advanced Cardiac Life Support (ACLS)	Advanced Cardiac Life Support (ACLS)	Health care providers in contact with adults at risk for cardiovascular emergencies	Use of monitor/defibrillators, transcutaneous pacing, advanced airway management skills, end-tidal carbon dioxide detection, basic EKG interpretation, identification and treatment of EKG rhythm changes, initiation of IV access and administration of emergency medications using preferred routes	Lecture, small group discussion, case-based scenarios with instructor feedback, learning by doing	Annotated written exam, with remediation as needed; evaluation of psychomotor skills

Continued on following page

American Heart Association Programs (Continued)

COURSE	MANUAL NEEDED	TARGET AUDIENCE	SKILLS LEARNED	EDUCATIONAL APPROACH	TESTING METHOD
Advanced Çardiac Life Support–Experienced Provider Program	Advanced Cardiac Life Support–Experienced Providers	Health care providers who routinely perform resuscitation as part of their job	Renewal course designed for experienced providers; covers all standard ACLS skills plus electrolyte abnormalities, cardiovascular-challenges, and environmental/toxicologic emergencies	Case-based, hands-on instruction with small group discussions and limited lecture	Annotated written exam and skills station
Neonatal Advanced Life Support (NALS)	Provider Manual for Neonatal Advanced Life Support	Health care providers who care for neonates or pregnant women	Skills needed for neonatal resuscitation, advanced airway management, CPR, ethical issues, and prevention of hypothermia	Case scenarios, limited lecture, and small group discussion	Annotated written exam and skills practice/evaluation

3. Do other organizations offer similar life support programs?

Yes. Perhaps the most widely known is the American Red Cross. Both AHA and Red Cross courses have been developed using the recommendations from the Emergency Care Committees. Consequently, the requirements and skills are quite similar. Perhaps the greatest difference between the two is that the Red Cross offers a wider variety of courses, including workplace safety, pet first aid and CPR, sports training, injury control, and oxygen administration. The AHA is focused on prevention and care of heart disease.

The National Safety Council provides online, computer-based first aid and CPR courses. The American Environmental Health and Safety Organization teaches an abbreviated CPR program. In addition, many organizations integrate the components of each of the above into their programs. For example, Advanced Medical Life Support (AMLS) programs include the AHA care guidelines. Finally, some organizations have collaborated on the development of advanced programs. For example, the American Academy of Pediatrics and American Heart Association collaborated to develop the neonatal resuscitation guidelines.

4. What does AHA certification mean? Why is it important?

The intent of AHA courses is not to document minimal competency by caregivers but to provide education and training to people responding to cardiovascular emergencies. Over the years hospital accreditation agencies have mandated documentation of acceptable proficiencies. Hospital leaders discovered that AHA course completion cards were a good way to document that staff members were qualified to respond appropriately to cardiac events in the hospital.

Course completion cards simply indicate that the person has attended the entire course, demonstrated at teaching stations command of the AHA recommendations, adequately performed CPR, and attained a satisfactory score on the written exam. Each of these items may be performed in remediation. Course completion does not guarantee future action, nor does it qualify or authorize a person to perform any skills. It indicates only that the person is able to perform in a simulated environment.

5. The AHA discourages using "course completion" as a method of documenting minimal competencies. How can hospitals demonstrate that staff members have established a minimal competency in emergency cardiovascular care (ECC)?

This question is difficult to answer because each institution has to develop individual competency measurement systems. Each department's performance evaluations should include skill-oriented behavioral objectives. Leaders should make clear the required minimal competencies for their employees. Simply conducting a class is no longer a sufficient method to ensure competency.

Clinical staff must be able to demonstrate specific techniques associated with life-saving procedures. There is no guarantee that education will translate into competent care.

There are mechanisms other than course completion cards to document an employee's achievement of minimal standards. Most organizations have policies outlining what constitutes competent care. Such policies usually contain samples of how to document specific competencies. At one hospital, for example, employees must attend annual ACLS training and must participate in simulated cardiac arrests annually to be considered competent in resuscitative care. Skills fairs are held to provide these competencies. Employees can also document competency by being observed as they care for patients in the clinical setting. Employees who participate in a real cardiac arrest and in the postarrest critique satisfy the mandate for annual competency assessment. Some organizations use checklists indicating that employees perform the task regularly. The key is to document that someone routinely and regularly monitors an employee's competency. The more learning opportunities you provide, the more competent an employee becomes. The AHA educational offerings augment a competency assessment but do not meet the standard by themselves.

6. The AHA structure seems quite complex. Describe its hierarchy.

At the national level, many volunteers and staff members support the mission of the AHA to reduce disability and death from heart disease and stroke. They are responsible for preparation of scientific and educational guidelines as well as product development and marketing. The 47 regional offices in the United States promote the work of the AHA in that region and support local work. At the local level, the community training center (CTC) is responsible for organizing, sponsoring, and implementing courses.

Definitions of the AHA Administrative Levels

National Emergency Cardiovascular Care Committee: made up of volunteers with scientific, educational, business, and administrative expertise to guide and direct the emergency cardiovascular care program. Members develop training materials and coordinate activities of the training network. They also manage business for the association.

Regional committees: made up of volunteers with medical, educational, business, and administrative expertise who develop and implement regional strategies to accomplish the goals and objectives set forth by the National Emergency Cardiovascular Care Committee training program.

National faculty: made up of volunteers with medical/health care expertise who serve as communicators between the local emergency cardiovascular care committees and the National Emergency Cardiovascular Care Committee.

Regional faculty: assigned by the AHA to community training centers to serve as a resource. These volunteers are AHA instructors who are responsible for quality and assist local emergency cardiovascular care committees in activities for the chain of survival.

Course directors: appointed by the community training centers for ACLS and PALS. They are responsible for course content and faculty assignments. The course directors should have at least two years' experience as an instructor in their specific discipline and should have taught at least eight courses. Breakdowns of their responsibilities are as follows:

- Select the faculty for each course.
- Monitor educational presentations for appropriateness.
- Supervise and evaluate student performance for skill stations.
- Be available during the courses for student questions.
- Monitor instructor performance.

Instructor trainers: for BLS discipline only. These BLS instructors have been appointed by the AHA to educate and evaluate instructors. Their responsibilities are as follows:

- Train BLS instructors according to the AHA guidelines.
- Ensure that instructors are updated and current with AHA guidelines.
- Teach at least three BLS courses per year to maintain their certification as instructor trainers.

Continued on following page

Definitions of the AHA Administrative Levels (Continued)

Instructors: teach provider courses in one or any of the AHA provider courses in which they are certified (BLS, ACLS, PALS). Instructors ensure consistency and quality of courses. Their responsibilities are as follows:

- BLS instructors need to maintain current knowledge of the various provider courses.
- ACLS and PALS instructors need to maintain current knowledge of adult and pediatric emergency cardiovascular care.
- They need to train providers according to AHA guidelines, regardless of which discipline they teach.
- They must teach at least two courses per year to maintain their certification.
- They must send all appropriate paperwork, such as course rosters and instructor status, to the community training center with which they are affiliated.
- No instructor can teach an AHA-sponsored course unless he or she is affiliated with an approved community training center.

Providers: the foundation of the AHA Emergency Cardiovascular Care program. Providers have successfully completed an approved AHA course for both theory and clinical skills in one of the disciplines.

7. What are the characteristics and skills of a good instructor?

Every instructor displays an individual personality, but the most effective instructors have certain similarities. They have taught the course before and have an understanding of the materials as well as the format. Unfortunately, expertise does not automatically make one a good teacher. All of us have taken classes from knowledgeable colleagues who lacked the ability to relay the information to students or were ineffective in classroom management.

In general, the best instructors possess good communication skills; have knowledge of the subject matter, a positive attitude, patience, empathy, and flexibility; and serve as role models by displaying professional behavior. In selecting faculty, you want someone who will be supportive of peers, staff, and participants. An enthusiastic, motivated, positive instructor who is genuinely concerned about his students makes a wonderful addition to the team. Tactfulness, friendliness, and professionalism in interactions are also positive qualities for providing constructive feedback to students.

The best instructors have realistic expectations and understanding of learners' needs and the ability to adapt their instruction to the experience levels and skill development of their students. They continuously consider the learners' perspective and adapt their teaching to meet student expectations. They are committed to ensuring that students receive the required instruction. Enthusiastic delivery is most effective at motivating student learning.

8. What procedures work well for recruiting high-quality instructors for life support classes?

Perhaps the most important point is to be constantly on the lookout for talented instructors. Observe instructors in practice. If they are respected and seem to demonstrate the qualities listed above, consider having them do a lecture or a skills station at an upcoming class. This approach allows you to evaluate their teaching skills. Many of the characteristics listed above are personality characteristics that are difficult to teach. It is far easier to teach someone how to teach or how to manage the classroom than it is to teach someone enthusiasm for the subject matter, empathy for students, or great communication skills. For this reason, do not rule out candidates because they have little or no experience; instead, mentor them to become great teachers.

Recruitment should include advertising the need for instructors. Seek manager and peer suggestions for potential instructors. An AHA life support course provides a solid structure for someone who is interested in teaching.

Part of the recruitment process involves working closely with people to accommodate their needs. Scheduling sessions around their work schedules and arranging for lunches to be served helps recruit and retain high quality instructors. Policies regarding payment for instructors vary, but instructors are more likely to give up a free weekend if they are rewarded financially for their effort. In addition, do not rule out community laypersons as instructors. Basic life support classes can be taught by nonmedical providers, many of who are enthusiastic and willing to teach in a variety of settings. This strategy frees health care providers to teach advanced courses in the health care setting.

9. How do I become an AHA Instructor?

Following are some of the prerequisites for taking an AHA instructor course:

- Present a current AHA provider completion card for the course you wish to teach.
- Present a letter from an affiliate/regional or course faculty member recommending that you become an instructor (not needed for Basic Life Support (BLS) instructors).
- Present a letter from a CTC coordinator indicating that the CTC will accept you as an instructor.
- Demonstrate a willingness and desire to teach in accordance with the scientific and program guidelines of the AHA.
- Each candidate must make a commitment to teach 2 courses per year according to AHA guidelines.

The requirements for becoming a Red Cross instructor are similar.

10. We use our instructors a lot. How can I help prevent burn-out?

Instructor burn-out is always a possibility, especially when the pool of qualified instructors is limited. An effective retention program is critical to success. It is wise to have a group of instructors to draw from rather than always relying on the same people. The number of courses offered by your facility every year should determine how many instructors you need. For best results, you should maintain 6–8 instructors for each program, depending on the number of participants. Encourage instructors to share topics, and avoid assigning them the same presentation or skills station at each class. Varying responsibilities and audiences helps prevent burn-out. For example, in one course, enlist an instructor's help to present a lecture portion. In the next course, the same instructor may coach a clinical skills station. The exception to this strategy is the instructor who does a superior job with a specific topic and enjoys presenting the information. Encourage instructors to teach lay people as well as experts on a rotating basis. When instructors are expected to provide a variety of presentations to a variety of people, they remain well rounded on all aspects of the program, and their work is more enjoyable.

11. Are there any other ways to retain instructors?

Instructors have identified the following factors as important reasons for continuing to teach life support programs. Your retention plan should focus on these issues.

- Good pay. Instructors want to be rewarded for what they know.
- Flexible schedule. Making the schedule convenient for educators is critical. Alternate weekend courses, evening courses, and weekday courses to achieve the maximal instructor participation.
- Administrative support. Adjust work schedules and arrange for relief coverage while an instructor is teaching. Provide administrative help so that classes run smoothly (e.g., enough supplies and copies).
- Recognition and feedback. Instructors want recognition for sharing their knowledge. They want to feel appreciated and valued.
- Participation in planning. Instructors want to have input in program planning and evaluation process. Once their ideas have been suggested, every effort should be made to implement them.
- Community service. Instructors believe that they are giving back to the community and providing a valuable service.

A key component to retaining high-quality instructors rests with the relationship between staff education leaders and assisting instructors. Staff educators should work diligently to build relationships with current and potential instructors by accommodating their needs and providing plenty of communication and support.

12. How do instructors stay current?

AHA instructors, whether teaching PALS, ACLS, or BLS, must demonstrate an understanding of the most recent guidelines. Attendance at an instructor renewal course can accomplish this goal. The following requirements also need to be completed:

- Demonstrate various psychomotor skills on a mannequin under the observation and supervision of a course faculty member.
- Maintain current status as a provider in the discipline that they are teaching.
- Achieve a satisfactory score on the instructor's written exam.
- Provide evidence of having taught two provider courses in the previous two years.

Some organizations offer AHA instructors continuing education opportunities through attendance at conferences. The AHA provides instructors with free online access to high-quality journals (www.currentsonline.com). In addition, many instructors have found valuable educational resources by surfing the Internet.

A structured evaluation plan for all instructors is necessary to ensure high-quality programs. Offer constructive peer critique, and provide frequent and regular feedback about how to improve presentations. In addition, students' course evaluations provide valuable data about instructors. At one facility, all of the faculty get together during lunches and have active and lively discussions about program improvement strategies. Another enjoyable option is to trade instructors with nearby training sites. This strategy allows instructors to learn new techniques, meet new people, and brainstorm about opportunities to improve their own programs.

13. What do you do with instructors who fail to maintain their teaching skills?

All instructors are mandated by AHA guidelines to play an active role in at least two courses per year. By meeting this guideline, they maintain their instructorship. If they do not meet this requirement, they can no longer instruct AHA courses unless they begin the renewal process for instructorship.

However, simply teaching two courses may not result in acceptable teaching skills. Instructors can be counseled about how to improve their teaching. Sometimes the course planners have to take a creative approach. During one recent course, an instructor struggled through a small group lecture but did an excellent job with students at the remediation station. Course planners can capitalize on each team member's strengths to put together a high-quality program.

14. How are AHA courses designed and set up?

One of the most exciting changes in the new AHA curricula is the ability for coordinators to set up programs that best meet the needs of their participants. The educational design of the courses includes large group interactive discussions, small group interactive discussions, discussion integrated with skills stations, video-mediated instruction, peer instruction, and slide-based lectures with interactive discussion. Regardless of the teaching method, most content is presented in a case scenario format.

Factors influencing course set up include availability of equipment, setting, number of instructors available to help, and skill level of people available to help. In addition, course planners should evaluate carefully the skill level of the participants. In its instructor manuals, the AHA provides a variety of course design options for all levels of courses. Each course includes a combination of skills practice and interactive discussion.

15. Much of the set up for AHA courses is based on changes made during the 2000 Emergency Cardiovascular Care Conference. Which of these changes are important for me to know?

Many experts agree that the following changes to the 2000 guidelines are the most significant:

CHANGE	SIGNIFICANCE
Move to an international, evidence-based approach	Experts all over the world are working on innovative methods for the treatment of cardiovascular emergencies. This movement will stimulate high-quality research and ensure that all future changes are safe, appropriate, and efficacious. Changes in the AHA guidelines will continue to be rapid and dynamic.
Simplification and brevity	Perhaps the most significant change is a realization that simple steps are easier to learn and easier to perform. Shortening BLS courses and decreasing the number of steps have resulted in increased ability to perform psychomotor skills adequately. Examples of simplification include: 1. Elimination of pulse check for lay rescuers. 2. Simplification in the management of foreign body removal. 3. Simplification of chest compressions, including finding landmarks and standardizing rates of compression. 4. Promoting easier-to-use airway adjuncts.
Promoting the use of adult learning principles	The new instructor course and recommended teaching methods are now consistent with the principles of how adults learn best.
Change in testing format/ promoting of remediation for students	Although controversial, the elimination of pass/fail criteria will have a huge impact on health care facilities' documentation of minimal competencies for staff. Remediation allows all individuals to succeed. Annotated written exams will allow students to learn from their mistakes.
Early defibrillation	Years of AHA training have failed to improve significantly the survival rates of sudden cardiac arrest. Promoting early defibrillation in a variety of settings by non–health care providers (e.g., police) will have a positive effect on mortality rates.
Guidelines contain medications used successfully in other areas	Guidelines recommend medications and techniques that have been used successfully in other countries areas for years (specifically, vasopressin and amiodarone). Other new treatment options will quickly emerge because of the international focus.
Refocus on acute coronary syndromes	Treatment proposals for acute coronary syndromes focus on prevention of tissue damage. This focus is important because it signifies a subtle change in philosophy—the shift to prevention and early treatment.
Friendlier environment	The courses have become much more user-friendly and less stressful. Teachers and students work collaboratively to reach the overall program goals.

16. I have been an instructor for many years. Do I have to take a new instructor course to implement the new AHA changes?

Currently the AHA mandates that current instructors complete a "rollout" program, which involves reviewing and practicing the recommended guidelines. The update takes about 4 hours per discipline. New skills are introduced that you will be expected to demonstrate.

17. Many of the instructors in my CTC are struggling with the new style of the AHA courses. What should I do?

The change in philosophy of the new AHA courses may require you to consider scheduling and organizing an instructor course. The newly developed instructor courses focus on adult learning principles and evidence-based learning. For most instructors, reviewing these principles will prove invaluable. The approach to teaching is different. Students are partners in the learning process. Testing is more instructional than evaluative. The learning environment is expected to be more relaxed. Even the experienced faculty person will benefit from a review of the new expectations. Providing practice time and allowing instructors to provide feedback to "mock" students and "student-teaching" in small groups will build confidence.

18. What are the steps for teaching students complex psychomotor skills?

Whether done live or by video, the AHA approach is as follows:

- **Instructor talk-through:** First the instructor provides a step-by-step description of the procedure in a small group environment (4–6 students).
- **Learner talk-through:** The participants are then asked to describe their basic understanding of the procedure.
- **First instructor demonstration:** Next the instructor provides a slow demonstration of the procedure with commentary about each step.
- **Second instructor demonstration:** The instructor demonstrates the procedure in real time with no commentary.
- **Learner walk-through:** The learners perform the procedures slowly under direct supervision of the instructor and group members. Learners describe what they are doing while doing it. Verbalization improves retention, as another sense is stimulated.
- **Ongoing feedback:** The instructor provides immediate feedback when an error is made.
- **Learner performance:** The learner performs the procedure at a real-time pace with no commentary.[7]

19. How do you prepare students at all levels (ACLS, PALS, NALS, BLS) for each course?

Properly preparing students before the start of any course is important to the overall success of the program. One of the first steps is to provide students with the text or manual at least 4 weeks before the course begins. For advanced life support courses, it is also helpful if you can provide participants with a folder full of additional information, such as an outline of the curriculum and copies of articles related to the subject. Provide participants with a pretest. Some instructors also provide students with a contact person to answer questions before the start of the program. Providing this information serves to ease the participants' anxiety.

Many facilities now offer optional precourse classes that provide first-time participants with an excellent foundation in the materials and hands-on skills needed for the various stations. These classes are helpful for those participants who want a good review, especially in areas that they do not often use as part of their job. This approach also provides an opportunity for instructors to prepare their own presentations for the actual course. Study guides, video series, computer programs, and board games are also helpful for preparing students. However, the simplification of the new AHA programs should permit most participants to be successful simply by reading the text before the program begins.

20. What are the advantages and disadvantages of case-based, small-group learning?

Case scenarios, case studies, and problem-based learning strategies have been used successfully in many disciplines for years. A case-based scenario allows the student to relate or identify with various situations from their own personnel experiences. When students are able to relate to these presentations, they tend to retain and recall more of the information. This method simulates critical thinking and problem-solving skills. Typical lecture material can be presented in a more practical, relevant context. Critical analysis of patient conditions can be done in a safe environment without the threat of endangering a patient. Case-based techniques are especially good for adult learners who desire peer interaction, support for prior experiences, and validation of thinking process.

Case-based learning is most effective when used with situations that require application; it is not as useful for relaying data or facts. Students must have a certain foundation of knowledge before they can solve a case study correctly. Teachers must be skilled in questioning techniques and feedback. Working through the case study questions requires participants to use teaching aids such as charts, notes, texts, or algorithms.

21. How can I teach effectively using the case-study approach?

The AHA cases build on one another and may be combined to ensure that students are able to accomplish the terminal objectives of the program. Encourage students to assume different roles during the cases (e.g., team leader, skill performer, evaluator). This strategy makes it more difficult for participants to assume a passive role in the learning process. Although it may be initially uncomfortable for some, studies have demonstrated that most adults prefer this learning method.

In addition, instructors should develop simple questions to stimulate small group discussion during the case scenario. Critical actions, relevant teaching points, and flexibility in instruction are crucial to the success of the case study. For example, if the student chooses an unsafe medication in the treatment of dysrhythmias, stopping the case study to discuss the actions and consequences of the medication serves as a valuable teaching tool.

As students progress from simple to more complex case studies, add more problem-solving or technical components. Be sure that what is added is consistent with what students may encounter in their work environment. The more relevant the case, the more likely that students will be able to apply and recall its basic principles at a later date. It is important to use the scenario as a teaching method rather than simply as a case presentation.

22. Can students really learn better by watching a video?

The main reasons for using video-mediated instruction are the consistency of content delivery and reduction in time needed for demonstration. Reduced demonstration time permits increased time for hands-on practice. Video instruction provides a structured stimulus for specific viewer responses, which may include development of a skill, change in behavior, or greater self-knowledge. The videotape technique effectively combines some aspects of feedback with modeling. The advantage of videotape is that the modeling is identical each time that it is presented. The instructor has the ability to stop the presentation at any time to enhance learning, to demonstrate important points, or to answer questions. For AHA programs, the use of videotape helps ensure that instructors stay on topic and do not provide information beyond the scope of the program.

Videotape technology alone, however, does not lead to improved learning. Learner readiness, specific focus, teacher comments, and a supportive environment are important to the successful use of videotape. Some seasoned AHA instructors have resisted a move to videotape, indicating that soon we will not need teachers anymore if leaders continue to replace them with technology. Empirical studies, however, demonstrate that students who are taught the new program with this method are more likely to retain skills and knowledge. It is a well-documented fact that the more senses that are stimulated during the learning process, the greater the learning. Video alone, however, is not effective for presenting material. Instructor interaction and feedback are critical to student success.

23. It is sometimes difficult to teach basic CPR to an expert provider and advanced ACLS skills to a novice with no other experience. How can instructors adjust the AHA standards for providers at different levels?

Depending on the situation, you may want to be selective in setting up your groups. You do not want your students to feel uncomfortable or intimated by other students. When basic courses include health care professionals, you need to stress the importance of the basics as a part of accepted standard of care. Give them the necessary information and performance skills based on AHA guidelines. Emphasize the fact that students must meet and perform at these standards to receive a course completion card. Any student who wishes to proceed to the advanced courses offered by AHA (ACLS and PALS) must have a completion card from the basic course.

When dealing with a participant who has had little exposure or experience with advanced skills, you may need to provide preparation classes to establish a sound foundation before the program even starts. This approach prevents the student from struggling through the course and feeling out of place among participants who may be more experienced. Instructors should be prepared to take every step possible to make courses rewarding for all participants. This goal may involve developing a course specifically for advanced providers or a course designed specifically for novices.

24. What creative strategies have been used to present the course content?

Certainly keeping the student interested and motivated is always a challenge, especially if the participant has been through the course several times in the past. Try to keep participants as involved as possible by asking questions or having them perform procedures. The more interactive the course, the more fun participants will have in learning the materials. Some instructors have made their presentation into the form of a game show in which they cover a topic and then have a panel whose members answer questions on the topic just presented.

25. What are my options for facilitating learning of skills by people with disabilities?

Each community training center is responsible for complying with all applicable laws, rules, and regulations, including the Americans with Disabilities Act (ADA). The AHA takes a strong stand against changes or deletions of items set in the core curriculum and manual. Any change is considered a fundamental change to the manual and may not be made in a course for which an AHA course completion card is issued. Individual instructors or community training centers must determine on their own what accommodations must be made to comply with the ADA. For example, hearing-impaired students can be accommodated by using a sign language interpreter. There are ways in which you can communicate with such persons so that they are able to perform the skills necessary to complete the course. Any person who is able to demonstrate performance of the skills required by the AHA and to pass the written exam will receive a course completion card. At times such situations may challenge the instructor's imagination, creativity, and teaching skills. However, experience has shown that AHA courses can be taught to most people with disabilities, especially if instructors elicit the help of family members or friends.

26. What resources are available to assist me in planning a course with the new changes?

Along with release of the 2000 education recommendations, the AHA has published many tools to assist regional faculty and training centers in program planning and organization. Instructor manuals, tool kits, slides, and supplies are available through several different companies, all of which provide catalogues with substantial selection options:

- Channing L. Bete Company (200 State Road, South Deerfield, MA 01371, 1-800-611-6083)
- Laerdal Medical Corporation (167 Myers Corners Road, PO Box 1840, Wappingers Falls, NY 12590, 1-800-562-4242)
- WorldPoint ECC, Inc. (151 S. Pfingsten Rd., Suite E, Deerfield, IL, 60015, 1-888-322-8350)
- CurrentsOnLine.Com, Inc. (United States and international guidelines 2000 on CD-ROM only; 25700 I-45 North, Suite 117, Spring, TX 77386, 1-281-419-8238)
- Lippincott Williams & Wilkins (351 West Camden Street, Baltimore, MD 21201, 1-800-638-3030; international phone, 1-301-223-2300)

The AHA website is extremely useful in providing answers to common questions. Browsers can access instructional material, including AHA publications (e.g., *Circulation* and *Currents*) and links to dozens of other useful, free resources. The current website providing assistance to instructors can be found at www.cpr-ecc.org/instructors/instructmenu.htm. You can also access the AHA home page at www.cpr-ecc.org/courses.html.

Your most useful resource may be your regional faculty member, who can answer questions and find materials. You can reach your Regional ECC Service Center at 1-888-277-5463.

Red Cross resources can be accessed by contacting your local American Red Cross chapter or on-line at www.redcross.org.

27. What creative ways have been used to secure the training equipment needed for courses?

In most facilities, the education department or training office generally has most of the equipment necessary for life support courses. Occasionally, however, specialty equipment may not be readily available. When searching for equipment, do not overlook organizations such as ambulance services or the state emergency medical service (EMS) office. They are often willing to allow the use of their equipment. Their personnel also may require the type of training that you offer. You also may be able to borrow equipment from inpatient hospital units. Manufacturers are often willing to donate equipment that will be used for training purposes. For example, one program recently secured expensive supplies from a manufacturer because the packages had been damaged and the contents were no longer sterile.

28. How do you evaluate the success of AHA courses? What other quality assurance or continuous quality improvement criteria does AHA mandate?

There are several ways to evaluate a course. In general, the best method is to calculate the number of participants who successfully complete both the written exam and skills stations. Participant evaluations are also extremely important in assisting to determine the effectiveness of the instructors. Suggestions made by participants for the improvement of any course should be taken seriously. Quality assurance is an important part of determining the success of existing or future courses. The AHA states that the community training center is solely responsible for the quality of the programs that it offers and compliance with policies and guidelines. Every course should be evaluated to determine whether it has met all of the standards according to AHA guidelines. The results can be useful in determining whether the instructor has met the needs of the participants.

29. What record keeping is required by the training center?

Several years ago, the AHA established community training centers. The purpose was to solidify local control for instructors and courses. The community training center coordinator is a liaison to the AHA. Coordinators are responsible for the following:

- **All record keeping.** Completed activity reports of each center are sent to the AHA's main office twice a year. Other areas of record-keeping responsibilities are issuing course completion cards, maintenance of course rosters, and documentation of administrative actions, quality assurance reports, and student evaluations.
- **Updating instructors** affiliated with the training center with the latest information on AHA courses, science guidelines, policies, and procedures. An updated instructor list must be maintained, along with evidence of the completion of instructor requirements. These records are kept for every discipline level (BLS, ACLS, and PALS) that the training center provides.

For American Red Cross courses, usually the local agency takes care of all record-keeping requirements for the instructor.

30. Which AHA courses are available online or via the computer?

A new computer version of BLS and ACLS, available through Laerdol Medical Corporation, has been approved by the AHA. The interactive learning system, called Heartcode, is a computer-based, self-learning program. It is not available via the Internet. Although the package is not inexpensive, the cost per participant is about $100. Heartcode software comes preloaded on either a desktop or laptop computer. A mannequin head outfitted with sensors connects to the computer to assess intubation skills for ACLS participants. Sensorized adult and infant mannequins accompany the BLS package.

ACLS students practice and are evaluated in a series of video scenarios, rhythm recognition exercises, a written exam, and an interactive MegaCode simulation. BLS students practice and are evaluated in adult and infant CPR, participate in simulated AED scenarios, and complete a written exam. After successful completion, each participant receives an AHA course completion or renewal card.

31. What are the advantages and disadvantages of computer-based BLS or ACLS?

The computer version of BLS/ACLS can provide a cost-effective method for educating staff. Students can complete the program at their own pace and with greater flexibility in scheduling than traditional instructor-led courses offer. The computer can be available 24 hours/day. The system bookmarks a student's progress, allowing frequent starts and stops. The system is also fun to use. In addition, the computer lessons can be used for teaching. For example, if you are teaching a rhythm recognition course, the rhythm strips can be projected using an LCD panel.

Obviously, independent computer learning is not for everyone, especially with content that is so important (and stressful to some students). The computer version is definitely programmed in a linear fashion, which can prove frustrating to a nurse who has learned a multitask approach. For example, if the nurse tells the computer to intubate the patient, the nurse must finish all tasks related to intubation before starting an IV line. The computer will dock points if the nurse tries to insert the IV before listening to lung sounds, even though in a real-life code these tasks are done simultaneously.

Finding a convenient, secure location can be difficult. A great deal of planning needs to go into the implementation of the Heartcode program to ensure its success.

CONTROVERSY

32. Should the pass-fail system be maintained or eliminated?

The use of AHA programs to test for competency distorts their educational mission. The new ACLS guidelines no longer require a minimal score to pass, and all participants do not have to achieve the same competency. Students who do not initially meet the minimal competency are remediated until they can pass. Experienced instructors have asked: "Doesn't this approach dilute the quality of education? Why should testing occur, if the written test has no meaning? How can learning occur if we are teaching simply to get students to pass the test?"

Arguments for maintaining the pass-fail system: Opponents of the recent change argue that possession of an ACLS card may no longer have any meaning. It does not matter how well or how poorly students perform on the written exam, nor does it matter how proficiently they act in the case scenarios. All students pass. Some argue that testing under the new guidelines serves only to assist in program evaluation. Because many employers continue to require an ACLS card, it is still expected that course completion indicates an ability to perform at a minimal standard. In addition, the legal benchmark for the standard of care for patients in cardiac arrest has traditionally been the AHA guidelines. Hospital performance improvement committees compare the care provided during cardiac arrests to the AHA algorithms. Therefore, professionals are held to this standard, even if the AHA does not want to consider the guidelines as national standards. In fact, they were built on *international consensus* that the recommendations are scientifically supported and evidence-based. As such they represent the minimal accepted standard of care. Participants should be able to pass the test independently before they receive a card. Only then can minimal competency be established. Because training centers cannot deviate from the AHA guidelines, people employed in areas requiring routine competency assessments must continue to demonstrate that they can appropriately respond in an emergency. Some hospital administrators need to seek alternative methods or courses to determine whether their staff can perform in a cardiovascular emergency.

Arguments for eliminating the pass-fail system: The goal should be to help all learners, regardless of ability. The AHA states that the object of is courses is *not* to ensure that all participants, with differing backgrounds and resuscitation roles, achieve the same level of knowledge and skill. The goal is simply to educate team members so that they are better prepared to perform appropriately in a cardiovascular emergency. The fear and anxiety of failing a course serve as a barrier to learning. Now students go into a program knowing that they will pass; they are internally motivated to learn what they need for their particular work role. Historically, personality conflicts with instructors and intimidation influenced whether a participant passed. Perhaps the most compelling argument for eliminating the pass-fail component rests with the fact that participants, whether certified or not, go to their work setting and apply what has been learned in the class. When faced with a cardiac arrest, a health care worker is still required to respond, whether or not they passed an AHA course. Thus, the goal should be to teach in a manner that encourages students to retain as much as possible from the class. Exams that are instructive instead of evaluative promote this concept. Participants are now remediated to the point that they can perform safely and appropriately in an emergency situation. In addition, development of explicit passing criteria for hands-on skills has been unsuccessful at the national level. In fact, there is no established national minimal competency or standard for the performance of skills. Rather than failing a student, the instructor assists him or her, by whatever means necessary, to ensure success. For students who truly are not motivated to succeed, the AHA criteria still dictate that they not receive a course completion card.

BIBLIOGRAPHY

1. American Heart Association: Community Training Center Administrative Manual. Dallas, American Heart Association, 1997.
2. American Red Cross. Instructors Corner On Line. Available at www.redcross.org/services/hss/resources/instructors.html, 2001.
3. Aufderheid TP, Stapleton ER, Hazinski MF (eds): Instructor's Manual—Heart Saver & AED. Dallas, American Heart Association. 1998.
4 Aufderheidec TP, Stapleton ER: American Heart Association, Instructor's Manual, Basic Life Support. Dallas, American Heart Association, 2000.
5. Bastable SB: Nurse as Educator: Principles of Teaching and Learning. Sudbury, MA, Jones & Bartlett. 1997.
6. Billi JE: Education in adult Advanced Cardiac Life Support training programs: Changing the paradigm. Ann Emerg Med 22:475–483, 1993.
7. Cummings RO, Hazinski, MF (eds): Guidelines 2000 for cardiopulmonary resuscitation and emergency cardiovascular aare: An international consensus on science. Circulation 102:8, 2000.
8. Cummings RO: Instructor's Manual—Advanced Cardiovascular Life Support. Dallas, American Heart Association, 2001.
9. Newell LD: Bringing 'em back: Resuscitation through the years. Every Second Counts Jan/Feb:10–14, 2001.

22. CLINICAL LADDERS

Connie H. *Gutshall*, MS, RN, CNA, *and Kristen* L. *O'Shea*, MS, RN

1. What is a clinical ladder?

A clinical ladder is a career development program designed to recognize registered nursing practice at the bedside. It serves as a means for registered nurses to be promoted without going into a management or administrative position. Various levels can be built into a clinical ladder as defined by each hospital/system. Advancement from one level of the clinical ladder to the next usually results in a corresponding increase in pay and responsibilities.

2. Why is a clinical ladder needed?

Because of the current nursing shortage, it is imperative to keep competent, caring nurses at the bedside. The clinical ladder supports the value of hands-on care and at the same time promotes personal and professional growth. Because nursing recruitment and retention are at the forefront of the current human resource dilemma, the clinical ladder rewards nursing expertise and the willingness to learn and grow.

3. What is the first step in implementing a clinical ladder?

The real question is "How interested are the staff nurses in your institution in having a clinical ladder?" To answer this question, you need to ask the nurses. Various methods can be used to gather their opinions and ideas, including focus groups and surveys (see Chapter 8, questions 11 and 15). If interest is great enough, you should move on to the next step.

4. Why would a registered nurse (RN) oppose a clinical ladder?

You may be surprised to learn that some of the staff nurses at your hospital will not be interested in a clinical ladder. The important issues are awareness of opposition and use of change management skills to work through what may become a difficult process to implement. Below are some of the reasons nurses may not want a clinical ladder:

- Change
- More work
- More involvement
- Seniority valued over work quality
- Competition between nurses
- Insecurity
- Viewed as more bureaucracy
- Fear of losing pay

5. What are the major financial considerations in implementing a clinical ladder?

Financial constraint in the current health care market can be one of the stumbling blocks to implementation. Salary increases need to be budgeted. Staff involvement with education and projects increases time away from the bedside (your hospital may call it nonproductive or indirect time).

6. How can I sell the value of a clinical ladder to administration?

Selling the value of the ladder to administration and the board of your hospital is your next important step. Below are a few of the critical selling points:

- Recruitment and retention
- Contributions to patients, nursing unit, hospital, and community
- Rewards that stretch people to attain a higher level of expertise
- Promotion of staff education
- Enhancement of professional nursing as a career rather than a job
- Advancement of clinical and professional practice
- Recognition and reward
- Improvements in nursing staff morale and job satisfaction, which in turn improve productivity

7. What is the next step in developing a clinical ladder?

You should identify a team of people to develop and implement the clinical ladder program. The people on this team should include:

- Staff nurses from various units, service lines, shifts, and experience levels
- Managers from various specialties
- Nursing administration
- Human resources representative
- And, of course, you, the staff development educator

8. What should the team do first?

The team's first objective should be to identify the basic tenets of your ladder. These tenets describe the foundation on which your ladder will be built and should be based on the feedback of nurses and managers about what they want from the process. Some of the tenets to consider include the following:

- The ladder must be realistic, attainable, easily understood, and concise.
- Criteria for advancement must be measurable, objective, and evaluated against a standard.
- The ladder must be consistently applied across the system.
- Criteria must value the depth of clinical practice, not just seniority.
- Advancement must be aligned with the evaluation process.
- Flexibility must be built into the options for advancement.
- The ladder must allow movement up as well as down, based on performance.
- Expectations increase as the nurse advances up the ladder.

9. What are the next steps?

Several components need to be developed before the clinical ladder program is implemented. Obviously, the components are related to the process that you develop for the clinical ladder. General steps include the following:

1. Identify a process for advancement.
2. Develop a policy or guideline that describes the process.
3. Develop performance tools that differentiate the levels of clinical practice.
4. Design tools that enhance the process:
   - Checklists (for advancing nurses, managers, and interviewers)
   - Necessary forms (application, reminder notices, sample letters)
   - Educational materials/manuals (examples, written description, frequently asked questions)
5. Identify a transition/implementation plan
6. Develop a means of ongoing oversight of the program

A sample checklist for an advancing nurse can be found in Appendix A. This form also reflects the process of advancement at a hospital.

10. How do you determine the number of levels in a clinical ladder?

The number of levels in a clinical ladder varies from hospital to hospital. As you define roles and behaviors, certain threads begin to emerge. For example, you may begin to see a continuum from novice to expert. Or certain roles and responsibilities required by your institution as a nurse advances up the clinical ladder (e.g., acting as a resource or educator) may emerge. The number of levels becomes evident as you and the group work through the process of describing nursing practice. Do not predetermine the number of levels that you need; let the work of the group drive the outcome. Some clinical ladders have as few as two levels and others as many as six. Considerations include the following:

- Ability to define clearly the specific differences in clinical practice at each of the levels.
- Financial resources: What is the salary range under consideration for the ladder? Are the differences among the levels significant enough to warrant a different pay grade?
- Time constraints: The greater the number of levels, the more often you will need to meet for advancements. The entire process will require more time.

- Need to create specialty roles to enhance departmental goals. For example, if clinical nurse specialists are not available, some specialty areas may need nurses who perform roles as researchers or educators.

11. What types of nurses fit the criteria for advancement in a clinical ladder?

Your organization needs to determine which nurses are eligible to participate in the ladder. Be certain that you have identified where all of the nurses in your institution work and determine whether they are a part of the clinical ladder program. Nurses are everywhere in your hospital. You may decide that only full- or part-time nurses who work in the in-patient setting are part of the clinical ladder. Temporary or as-needed nurses may be excluded. This approach is common. Factors to consider in this decision are nurses who:

- Work on inpatient units
- Work weekends
- Work holidays
- Work rotating shifts
- Work on specialized units
- Work on call as required

The main focus for this program is to reward nurses at the bedside. Advanced practice nurses and nurses in administration are usually already at a higher salary or have the opportunity for higher pay overall. Including them in the clinical ladder can be a deterrent for clinicians who see their participation as a continuance of the usual hierarchy, with the clinical nurse once again at the lower end of the spectrum. Having a clinical ladder program strictly for staff nurses reinforces the importance that you place on their positions.

12. How does a clinical ladder relate to performance management?

The performance evaluation system and the clinical ladder are critically linked. As you create the criteria for each evaluation heading in the clinical ladder, you are essentially creating the evaluation tool for performance management. Behaviors and actions that are required for the clinical ladder become the mainstay of the evaluation.

13. What evaluation headings are common for nurses in a clinical ladder?

Your group needs to identify the key roles that a nurse performs at your hospital. The headings may vary, depending on the type of practice and the values of your nursing department.

Evaluation Headings

HOSPITAL A	HOSPITAL B	HOSPITAL C
Clinical practice	Clinical	Practitioner
Leadership	Educational	Educator
Professional development	Administrative	Consultant
Communication	Research	Researcher
		Administrator
		Leader

14. How should we operationalize the evaluation headings?

After you have defined the general headings, it is helpful to break your task force into small groups. The goal for each of the small groups is to define the specific behaviors for one of the evaluation areas. The group should refer to the literature and examples of other ladders. At this point, group members should describe carefully the preferred behaviors within the key area. They then need to begin to describe how nurses differ professionally within that key area (e.g., comparison of novice nurses, competent nurses, and expert nurses). The outcome will be performance evaluations for each level of the clinical ladder. It is helpful during this process to compare the evaluations of each levels side by side to ensure that performance expectations increase with each level.

15. What resources are available to help us?

- Obtain examples of current ladders from other institutions.
- Review the literature.

- Speak with other hospitals about their program.
- Go on site visits. Interaction with staff as well as nursing administration will give you a picture of how the program functions.
- Ask nurses who have worked in other institutions to share feedback about the positive and negative aspects of ladders with which they have been involved.
- Invite members of your human resources department to participate. They have extensive knowledge and experience in performance management issues.

16. How does a nurse advance up the clinical ladder?

This process is decided by you and your team. You need to define several key areas:

- How to evaluate a nurse's readiness to advance
- Time frames, including the experience needed for each level, how long before a new graduate nurse can apply, how to hire an experienced nurse into the clinical ladder, and amount of time required between advancements
- The step-by-step process for advancement
- Frequency of advancement (Is it offered only at certain times of the year or continuously?)
- Appeals process/demotion process

It is helpful to create a guideline or policy to communicate the process once you have defined these key areas.

17. What are the options for evaluating a nurse's readiness for advancement?

- Manager evaluation
- Peer evaluation
- Self-evaluation
- Exemplar submission
- Portfolio
- Interview by peers or management

Your team needs to determine what type(s) of evaluation will fit culturally within your hospital. Any combination of the above can be used. You may need to use several methods to provide the depth of information that you will need for evaluation.

18. What is an examplar?

An exemplar is a piece of writing that demonstrates application of nursing knowledge. An exemplar may showcase a particularly complex patient situation or a conflict resolution on the unit that required extraordinary leadership skills. Supporting documents can be included to show evidence of exemplary practice.

19. What should be included in a portfolio?

A portfolio is an accumulation and presentation of professional accomplishments. Included in the portfolio are evidence of attendance at educational offerings, outlines of programs or inservices that the candidate has presented, commendations, patient compliments, and competencies. A portfolio reflects how performance expectations are met or exceeded. Brooks and Madda provide a solid reference for portfolio development.[1]

20. What needs to be considered when peer interviews are used for evaluating readiness for clinical advancement?

Peer interviews can be a useful technique for evaluating readiness for advancement if the interviewers are prepared and trained in advance. One hospital advances nurses based on the decision of an advancement panel. The panel reviews peer, self, and manager evaluations as well as a submitted portfolio. Then the panel interviews the candidate, verifying information and exploring areas of potential weakness. The education of the staff on the panel is extremely important.

21. What topics should be included in the education of peer interviewers?

- In-depth information about the clinical ladder advancement process (interviewers may be helpful in educating others and serve as proponents of the ladder)
- Clear descriptions of expectations and behaviors of the various levels of the clinical ladder
- Critical issues such as confidentiality

- Decision-making model (e.g., consensus or majority vote)
- How to create a supportive environment for a nervous interviewee
- How to prepare and ask open-ended questions
- How to ask meaningful follow-up questions

22. How should staff be educated about the clinical ladder during implementation?

The success of clinical ladder implementation hinges on clear communication and education that support the process. Information should be provided using a variety of methods, such as general sessions, staff meetings, and written communication. The following considerations should be kept in mind:

- Meetings must be held on different days of the week and during different shifts to reach all staff.
- Forums at which staff can ask questions, raise doubts, and get answers help the program to go more smoothly.
- If your staff has e-mail, use it for announcements, changes, and reference.
- Use the traditional paper memo to announce the clinical ladder program to all staff nurses. Consider mailing it to their homes. This strategy makes a clear statement about the importance of the information.
- Provide managers with clear scripts of information about the clinical ladder for staff meetings and other informal discussions. Make sure that important points are identified for easy reference.
- Consider creating a manual that contains information about the clinical ladder program, and make it available on every participating nursing unit.

The more communication venues utilized, the better.

23. What staff education/information is needed during the implementation of your clinical ladder?

- General process for advancement
- Descriptions of the various levels of the clinical ladder
- Information about the evaluation process
- Examples of how the process works for different types of employees (new, experienced, transferring)
- Examples of evaluation tools

In addition, if you have built such elements as portfolio development or exemplar writing into your evaluation methods, staff may need additional education and support about these topics. Education for peer interviewers is listed in question 20. Another potential area for education is how to write meaningful peer evaluations.

24. What other implications does the clinical ladder have for staff development educators?

As staff members become more involved in their own development as professionals, the need for additional educational offerings and more advanced educational offerings will increase. Staff may be interested in becoming involved in teaching such courses. As a nurse advances up the clinical ladder, he or she may need to build skills in areas such as facilitation of projects, meeting management, presentation skills, computer use, research, finance, and a host of other leadership development offerings.

Staff development educators also may become involved in career counseling and coaching. Helping nurses find and build on areas of strength is quite rewarding. A clinical ladder brings many positive opportunities for involvement by the staff development department.

25. How long will it take us to develop a clinical ladder program?

Like any group process, it will take longer than you expect. Development of a ladder with true input and clearly defined expectations may take from 1 year to 18 months. This period also includes a thorough educational process. One important element is to hold stakeholder meetings at which the ladder under development is presented to staff. The feedback will assist you in defining controversial or problematic areas. These meetings are also an opportunity to begin the change process for staff members still wary of the process.

26. How can I be sure that the clinical ladder program is applied consistently throughout the organization?

It is important that the clinical ladder program is applied consistently throughout your institution. Possible methods for addressing this issue include:

- Baseline education for everyone
- Oversight panel (group of stakeholders who meet monthly or regularly to continue to define and refine the ladder; include one member from each nursing department or service line)
- Panel chair meetings (so that chairs of the advancement interview panels can discuss issues)
- Administrative education, involvement, and support
- Appointment of a person to assist advancement panels or committees across the organization and to act as a resource, educator, and reliability anchor.

27. How should I evaluate the success of a clinical ladder program?

A clinical ladder program is an example of an initiative that requires all five levels of evaluation (see Chapter 17).

LEVEL OF EDUCATION	WHAT?	HOW?
1	Satisfaction	Evaluation by participants advancing on the clinical ladder Evaluation by members of the advancement committee (who need to collect issues to be resolved) Measure of satisfaction of nursing staff as a whole (may be part of an employee satisfaction survey)
2	Knowledge	Number of successful advancements per department
3	Application of knowledge	Quantify increased participation of staff in education, research, and performance improvement initiatives Measure of degree of increase in professionalism by means of an established tool
4	Impact	Number of nurses recruited Measure of retention statistics Productivity
5	Return on investment/ program evaluation	Calculate return on investment (ROI) Determine whether the programs is important enough to retain

28. When do we know that we are finished with the development of our clinical ladder?

One of the most common errors in a clinical ladder program is to underestimate the amount of time required for maintenance after the initial implementation.To sustain enthusiasm and uphold the tenets of the clinical ladder, you must view it as a continuous improvement process. Your clinical ladder will never be finished. You must build a system for continued oversight and progression of the process. Use of an oversight group that meets regularly is helpful.

29. For what functions is an oversight committee responsible?

- Ongoing communication (e-mail or regular newsletters)
- Maintaining consistency
- Keeping materials updated
- Updating the process to keep it in line with hospital, system, or practice changes
- Discussing and solving problems
- Acting as resources
- Evaluation

30. What other factors should be considered?

The ladder reflects institutional culture. Ensure that your task force "grows" its own program and does not simply adopt someone else's ladder. The performance expectations have to make sense to the staff; if you use someone else's expectations, you may not succeed in defining practice for your hospital.

Appendix A: Sample Clinical Ladder Checklist

Steps for application for the Clinical Practice Advancement Program

_____ 1. Review criteria for the level for which you are applying. Objectively and comprehensively evaluate your clinical practice, leadership, and communication abilities.

_____ 2. Optional step: Set up a meeting with your coach (nurse manager, clinical nurse specialist, CN3, clinical advancement panel member, etc.) to review your performance as it relates to the criteria for the level for which you are applying.

_____ 3. Based on the conversation with your coach, you may choose to spend additional time improving your performance and clinical practice, or you may choose to continue to step 4.

_____ 4. Set up a meeting with your nurse manager to review your performance evaluation, self-evaluation, and clinical practice as it relates to the criteria for the level for which you are applying.

_____ 5. Together with your nurse manager, complete your Letter of Intent to Advance and determine the five RNs for your peer review. Submit to the Chair of the Service Line Advancement Panel (by the first Monday of January, May, or September). Late submissions will not be accepted. You will receive confirmation of your application in 1 week. If you don't receive confirmation, please notify your panel chair.

_____ 6. Update your resume.

_____ 7. Update your portfolio by using the professional development checklist. Each item circled on the professional development checklist must have supporting documentation (e.g.., verification of completion of criteria form (VCC), letters of commendation, picture of bulletin board or poster).

_____ 8. Review your portfolio and resume with your nurse manager or chair of the Service Line Advancement Panel at least one month prior to submitting your portfolio.

_____ 9. Distribute the peer evaluations for the level of which you are advancing (CN2 or CN3) 1 month before the advancement to the five RNs listed on your Letter of Intent. Inform peers that upon completion, the evaluation must be returned to the chair of the Service Line Advancement Panel in a confidential envelope (by the first Monday of the month you are advancing).

_____ 10. Complete your self-evaluation using the criteria for the level which you are advancing (CN2 or CN3).

_____ 11. Submit your portfolio, self-evaluation, and resume to the Chair of the Service Line Advancement Panel by the first Monday of the month you are advancing. Late submissions will not advance.

_____ 12. Relax and remember to focus on your clinical practice and the contributions you make to our patients everyday.

BIBLIOGRAPHY

1. Brooks BA, Madda M: How to organize a professional portfolio for staff and career development. J Nurs Staff Devel 15:5–10, 1999.
2. Goodloe LR, et al: Clinical ladder to professional advancement program. J Nurs Admin 26(6):58–64, 1996.
3. Gustin TJ, et al: A clinical advancement program: Creating an environment for professional growth. J Nurs Admin 28(10):33–39, 1998.
4. Krugman M, et al: A clinical advancement program: evaluation 10 years of progressive change. J Nurs Admin 30:215–225, 2000.
5. Kruvutske ME, Fox DH: Creating a registered nurse advancement program that works. J Nurs Admin 26(11):17–22, 1996.

INDEX

Page numbers in **boldface type** indicate complete chapters.